ANTI-INFLAMM CORTISOL RESET DETOX DIET FOR WOMEN OVER 40

The Practical Guide with Quick & Easy Recipes to Sleep Better, Boost Energy, and Finally Flatten Your Belly

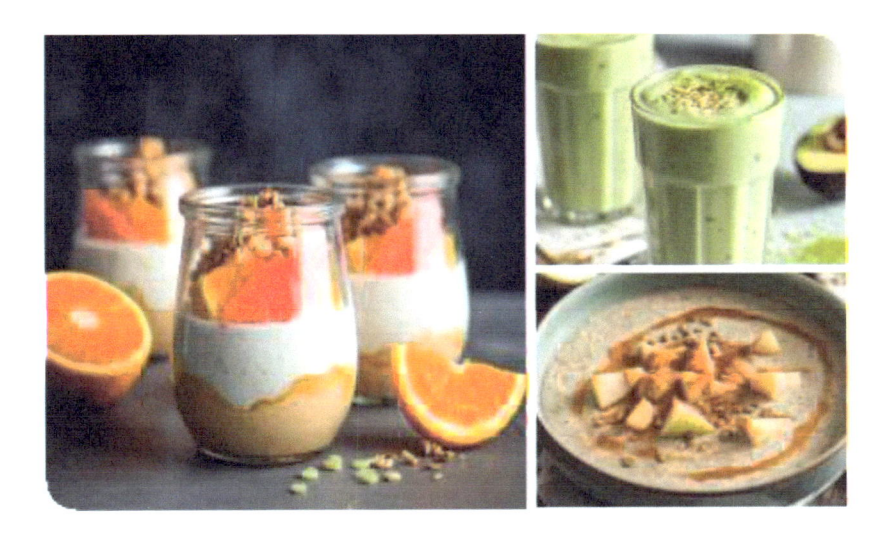

Author:
Dana Harvey

© 2025 Dana Harvey - **All Rights Reserved**

Anti-Inflammatory Cortisol Reset Detox Diet for Women Over 40.

The content of this book is provided with the intent to offer accurate and reliable information. However, by purchasing this book, you acknowledge that neither the publisher nor the author claim expertise in the topics discussed, and any advice or recommendations are provided solely for entertainment purposes. It is recommended that you consult with professionals as necessary before taking any action based on the content of this book.

This disclaimer is recognized as fair and valid by both the American Bar Association and the Committee of Publishers Association, and is legally binding across the United States.

Unauthorized transmission, duplication, or reproduction of any part of this work, whether electronic or printed, including the creation of secondary or tertiary copies, or recorded versions, is prohibited without the express written consent of the publisher. All rights not expressly granted are reserved.

The information presented in this book is deemed to be truthful and accurate. However, any negligence in the use or misuse of this information by the reader is their sole responsibility, and under no circumstances will the publisher or the author be liable for any consequences or damages that may arise from the use of this information.

Furthermore, the information contained in this book is intended solely for informational purposes and should be treated as such. No guarantees are made regarding the ongoing validity or quality of the information. Trademarks mentioned are used without permission and their inclusion does not constitute an endorsement by the trademark holder.

ISBN: 979-8-90046-820-4

Email: selfpublishing110186@gmail.com

TABLE OF CONTENTS

UNDERSTANDING CORTISOL AFTER 40 ----------- 6
- WHY STRESS HITS HARDER IN MIDLIFE ----------- 6
- CORTISOL, BELLY FAT, AND HORMONAL SHIFTS ----------- 7
- EVERYDAY CORTISOL TRIGGERS ----------- 8
- HIDDEN FOODS THAT KEEP YOU INFLAMED ----------- 8
- SUGAR, SEED OILS, AND PROCESSED FOOD OVERLOAD ----------- 10
- STRESS, SLEEP LOSS, AND EMOTIONAL EATING ----------- 12
- RESET FOUNDATIONS ----------- 14
- MANAGING INFLAMMATION AND CORTISOL THROUGH NUTRITION ----------- 14
- CHOOSING BETWEEN STANDARD, LOW-FODMAP, GENTLE ----------- 15
- LIFESTYLE HABITS THAT CALM CORTISOL ----------- 16
- SLEEP RITUALS THAT ACTUALLY WORK ----------- 16
- *Evening Sleep Ritual Checklist* ----------- 17
- GENTLE MOVEMENT VS. EXHAUSTIVE WORKOUTS ----------- 18

QUICK & EASY ANTI-INFLAMMATORY RECIPES ----------- 19
- ENERGIZING 10-MINUTE BREAKFASTS ----------- 20
- LUNCH BOWLS & WRAPS ----------- 25
- ONE-PAN 20-MINUTE DINNERS (5 RECIPES) ----------- 30
- NO-BAKE SNACKS & SWEET FIXES ----------- 36

ENERGIZING BREAKFASTS ----------- 41
- SMOOTHIE & SHAKE RECIPES ----------- 42
- EGG-BASED RECIPES ----------- 47
- GRAIN-FREE AND LOW-GRAIN RECIPES ----------- 52
- FAMILY-FRIENDLY GRAB-AND-GO: 5 RECIPES ----------- 57

SATISFYING LUNCHES ----------- 63
- FRESH SALADS AND NOURISH BOWLS ----------- 64
- HEARTY SOUPS & STEWS (5 RECIPES) ----------- 69
- PROTEIN-PACKED WRAPS & PLATES ----------- 75
- 5 LUNCHBOX RECIPES FOR BUSY DAYS ----------- 80

NOURISHING DINNERS ----------- 86
- SHEET PAN AND ONE-POT MEALS ----------- 87

- LEAN PROTEIN MAINS --- 92
- PLANT-BASED GENTLE OPTIONS --- 97

SNACKS, SIDES, AND LONG-TERM SUCCESS --- 101

- ANTI-INFLAMMATORY SNACK RECIPES --- 102
- SMART BEVERAGES & HEALING INFUSION RECIPES --- 107
- REINTRODUCING FOODS SAFELY --- 112
- 30-Day Cortisol Reset Meal Plan --- 114
- Conclusion --- 119

UNDERSTANDING CORTISOL AFTER 40

WHY STRESS HITS HARDER IN MIDLIFE

Tip

If you're struggling with morning fatigue or restless nights, try stepping outside for 10 minutes of natural light within an hour of waking. This simple habit helps reset your cortisol rhythm, supports better sleep, and can boost your mood. Pair it with a nourishing breakfast rich in fiber and healthy fats to further stabilize energy and reduce cravings. Small, consistent changes like these can make a big difference in how you feel each day.

As women enter midlife, physiological and lifestyle changes can broaden and intensify stress, with a key driver being the hormonal shift from declining **estrogen** and **progesterone**. These hormones help regulate mood, metabolism, and the body's stress response, and when their levels fall, **cortisol** — the main stress hormone — can lose its normal rhythm.

While some women experience dramatic changes, others may notice more subtle shifts. Cortisol normally peaks in the morning to support waking and then falls through the day; during midlife this pattern can flatten or invert, causing morning fatigue and increased nighttime restlessness.

Hormonal fluctuations also disrupt sleep, producing frequent awakenings or trouble falling asleep. Poor restorative sleep amplifies tension and creates a self-reinforcing cycle. **Metabolic flexibility** — the ability to switch efficiently between burning carbohydrates and fats — often declines with age, which can increase inflammation and make it harder to maintain a healthy weight, especially around the abdomen.

Life roles often change at this stage and can add pressure: many women balance caregiving for children and aging parents, face career stagnation, or shoulder financial strain. While these circumstances vary widely from person to person, these responsibilities tend to raise cortisol and contribute to visceral fat accumulation, stronger cravings, unstable blood sugar, and cognitive issues like *brain fog*.

Chronic stress commonly shows up as persistent abdominal weight gain, the typical 3 p.m. energy slump, and the frustrating combination of feeling wired yet tired at night. Other signs include anxiety, reduced libido, and joint discomfort. Though individual experiences differ, disruption of the cortisol curve can trigger a cascade of health problems, including increased abdominal fat that raises cardiovascular and diabetes

CORTISOL, BELLY FAT, AND HORMONAL SHIFTS

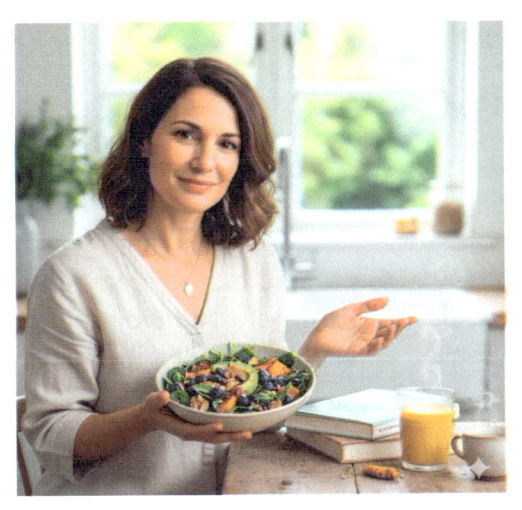

Chronic elevation of cortisol, the body's primary stress hormone, triggers metabolic changes that significantly affect women's health, particularly after **age 40.** When cortisol stimulates glucose production, sustained high levels prompt continuous glucose release and persistently elevated blood sugar.

This forces the pancreas to release more insulin, and prolonged elevation can lead to insulin resistance—a condition where cells become less responsive to insulin while excess glucose converts to fat, particularly visceral fat around the abdomen.

Visceral fat lies deeper within the abdominal cavity, surrounding vital organs. Unlike subcutaneous fat, this metabolically active tissue functions as an endocrine organ, releasing inflammatory cytokines including interleukin-6 (IL-6) and tumor necrosis factor-alpha (TNF-α).

These compounds promote chronic inflammation and interfere with insulin signaling, worsening insulin resistance and encouraging more visceral fat accumulation—creating a self-perpetuating cycle that increases risk of cardiovascular disease and **type 2 diabetes.**

Disrupted cortisol circadian rhythm intensifies this pattern. While cortisol typically peaks in the morning and declines throughout the day, chronic stress can elevate nighttime levels, increasing appetite for high-calorie foods and compromising sleep quality.

Poor sleep then affects hunger hormones ghrelin and leptin, causing stronger cravings and increased appetite, further contributing to visceral fat gain.

During **their 40s, women experience hormonal shifts that significantly affect this cortisol-insulin interplay**. Declining estrogen reduces insulin sensitivity, while falling progesterone—which supports stress resilience—increases perceived stress and vulnerability to elevated cortisol.

These changes can impair leptin sensitivity, increase hunger and cravings, and slow T4-to-T3 thyroid hormone conversion, potentially reducing metabolic rate.

During perimenopause, anovulatory cycles create erratic patterns that worsen symptoms like brain fog and favor abdominal fat gain. The hypothalamic-pituitary-adrenal (HPA) axis controlling stress response can become overactive, with chronic stress and hormonal shifts potentially dysregulating this system and elevating cortisol.

EVERYDAY CORTISOL TRIGGERS

HIDDEN FOODS THAT KEEP YOU INFLAMED

Many women over 40 choose "healthy" labeled foods without realizing some promote inflammation and disrupt cortisol balance. Identifying hidden culprits enables smarter eating choices.

Ultra-processed low-fat yogurts and snack bars appear healthier but manufacturers add carrageenan and **polysorbate-80** for texture and shelf life. Research suggests these additives harm gut microbiome and increase intestinal permeability, triggering systemic inflammation and affecting cortisol. Plain, full-fat yogurts without added sugars offer probiotics without inflammatory additives.

Seed oils like soy, corn, and canola in salad dressings and rotisserie chickens contain high omega-6 fatty acids. Excessive omega-6 relative to omega-3 may worsen inflammation. Extra-virgin olive or avocado oil provide anti-inflammatory monounsaturated fats.

Whole grain breads and tortillas provide fiber but gluten drives inflammation in people with celiac disease or sensitivity. Those sensitive might explore sourdough (fermentation reduces gluten) or gluten-free options from roots and tubers.

Flavored oat milks contain added sugars and oils promoting inflammation, spiking blood glucose, and contributing to insulin resistance. Unsweetened plant milks with minimal ingredients offer cleaner alternatives.

Deli meats contain nitrates and nitrites forming nitrosamines linked to inflammation and cancer risk. Minimally processed turkey or chicken without preservatives provides cleaner protein.

Artificial sweeteners like sucralose and aspartame in diet products may disturb gut bacteria, causing dysbiosis and inflammation. Natural sweeteners like stevia or monk fruit have less documented gut impact. High-fructose corn syrup in fitness drinks promotes liver fat accumulation and insulin resistance. Beverages without added sugars or water infused with fresh fruit offer better alternatives.

Light alcoholic seltzers disrupt sleep, raise inflammation, and disturb circadian rhythms. Sparkling water with citrus provides a noninflammatory option.
Nightshade vegetables contain solanine, potentially worsening joint pain in some people. Those with joint issues should track intake and watch symptoms.

High-histamine foods—leftovers, aged cheeses, kombucha—affect inflammation in people with histamine intolerance, causing headaches, anxiety, or sleep disruption. Fresh, minimally processed options may help manage symptoms.

Begin with a 10–14 day elimination phase removing common inflammatory triggers: seed oils, gluten, refined sugars, artificial sweeteners, emulsifiers, and high-histamine ferments and alcohol. Continue eating quality protein, fiber, and essential minerals to avoid nutrient gaps.

Daily record sleep latency, night awakenings, waist measurements, energy levels, food cravings, skin condition, joint pain, and mood. This log helps connect foods with symptoms, though individual responses vary.

After elimination, reintroduce one food category every three days. Note gastrointestinal upset, brain fog, anxiety spikes, rebound cravings, or post-meal heart rate rises over 10 bpm—these indicate sensitivity.

Stretch your budget with cost-effective anti-inflammatory options:
canned fish in water or olive oil for omega-3s bulk dry beans for fiber and protein frozen vegetables and berries retaining most nutrients

Choose pasture-raised eggs when possible; if budget-constrained, conventional eggs cooked in olive oil remain nutritious. Cook larger meat portions and freeze in single-use portions to limit histamine buildup.

Clear pantry of elimination-phase offenders and restock with extra-virgin olive oil, nuts and seeds, whole grains (quinoa, brown rice), and inflammation-reducing spices like turmeric and ginger.

SUGAR, SEED OILS, AND PROCESSED FOOD OVERLOAD

Tip

Batch-cooking proteins and roasting vegetables at the start of the week can be a game-changer for busy women. Prepping these basics ensures you always have healthy, anti-inflammatory options ready, making it easier to avoid processed foods and stick to your reset plan.

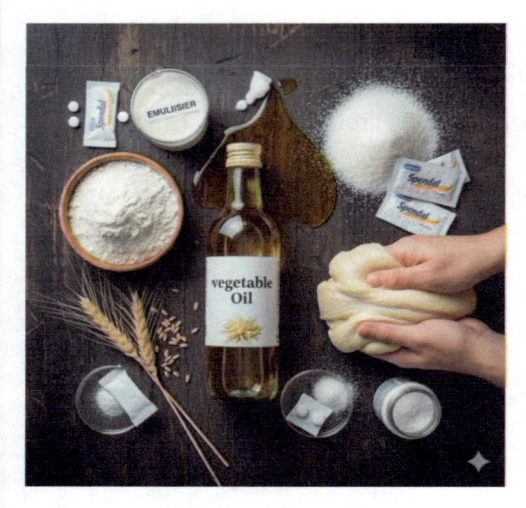

Resetting cortisol and cutting inflammation often begins with building an anti-inflammatory plate that outlines what to include and what to avoid—particularly added sugars and seed oils that tend to hide in processed foods. Many find success centering meals on specific macronutrient ratios and healthy fats to support hormonal balance and lower inflammation.

Consider aiming for **25–35 grams of protein per meal** from sources like eggs, poultry, fish, or plant-based options such as tofu and tempeh. A 3.5-ounce grilled chicken breast contains about 31 grams of protein, while a 4-ounce salmon fillet provides roughly 25 grams plus **omega-3s** that may help reduce inflammation.

Including at least **two cups of non-starchy vegetables per meal** can be beneficial. Vegetables such as broccoli, spinach, kale, and bell peppers supply vitamins, minerals, antioxidants, and fiber that research suggests fight inflammation. One cup of chopped broccoli has about 2.6 grams of fiber and plenty of vitamin C. Roasting these vegetables in 1–2 tablespoons of extra-virgin olive oil enhances flavor while adding monounsaturated fats that support heart health.

Adding slow-digesting carbohydrates like sweet potatoes, squash, and berries can supply nutrients and fiber without dramatically spiking blood sugar. A medium sweet potato contains about 4 grams of fiber and is rich in vitamin A; roasting or steaming these foods helps preserve nutrients and enhance flavor.

Many nutritionists recommend limiting added sugars to under **6 grams per serving** and no more than **24 grams per day**. Since sugar appears in many processed items, natural alternatives work well: *fresh fruit with cinnamon* or a small square of *100% cacao chocolate* provides antioxidants and satisfies sweet cravings without refined sugar.

Consider avoiding snacks and dressings made with seed oils (soybean, canola) that are high in omega-6s. Nuts, seeds, olives, or homemade vinaigrettes offer alternatives. For example, whisking olive oil with balsamic vinegar and a dash of mustard creates salad dressing, while air-popped popcorn drizzled with olive oil and sea salt provides a crunchy snack without processed oils.

Batch-cooking proteins and roasting vegetables ahead of time ensures healthy choices are ready and helps avoid impulsive processed-food picks.

Preparing grilled chicken or roasted chickpeas at the start of the week makes it easy to build quick salads or bowls.

Carrying "oil + protein" emergency kits for on-the-go meals—tuna packed in olive oil or single-serving nut butter packets—are portable options that help you skip fast food while maintaining balanced choices.

Transform your breakfast into a savory meal to cut back on processed items. Instead of sweet granola or bars, consider eating a nutrient-dense breakfast of **two scrambled eggs**, a handful of sautéed spinach, and **half an avocado**. That combination provides about 20 g of protein, 15 g of healthy fats, and 7 g of fiber, which may help keep you full and stabilize blood sugar to reduce mid-morning energy.

STRESS, SLEEP LOSS, AND EMOTIONAL EATING

To disrupt the stress-sleep-cortisol cycle, creating a structured daily routine with specific morning and evening practices can be helpful. Start your day with a **10–15 minute walk in natural light**; this simple activity exposes you to sunlight, which helps regulate circadian rhythm, and boosts serotonin to improve mood and reduce stress. While outdoor walking tends to be more effective since natural light works better than artificial light, sitting by a sunlit window can serve as an alternative when going outside isn't possible.

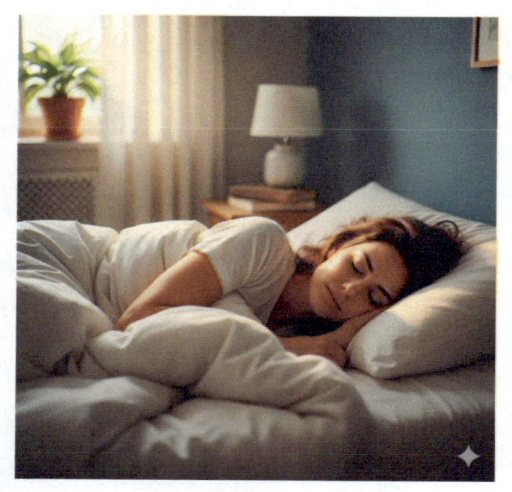

In the evening, consider using a **5–10 minute wind-down routine** to lower cortisol and increase sleep drive. Some people find success with **nasal breathing** (inhaling and exhaling through the nose) to promote relaxation, the **legs-up-the-wall pose** (lying on your back with legs vertical against a wall) to calm the nervous system, or the **4-7-8 breathing method**: inhale through the nose for *4 seconds*, hold for *7*, and exhale through the mouth for *8*; repeat six cycles.

Set a non-negotiable sleep window of **7.5–8.5 hours in bed** and maintain a consistent sleep schedule to support a healthy cortisol rhythm and make falling asleep and waking easier. Many experts suggest limiting caffeine after **12 p.m.**, since it can stay in your system and potentially disrupt sleep. Similarly, avoiding alcohol **3–4 hours before bedtime** may help, as it can fragment sleep and increase night wakings.

Creating a dim-light evening routine often improves sleep quality. After sunset, use blue-light filters on devices to reduce blue light that suppresses melatonin, and turn off electronics at least **60 minutes before bed** to allow your body to shift toward rest. A warm shower before bed can be beneficial because the following drop in body temperature signals it's time to sleep. Some people find **magnesium glycinate (200–400 mg)** in the evening supports relaxation, while others prefer an *Epsom-salt foot soak* for a similar calming effect.

Make your sleep environment restful by keeping the room cool (65–68°F) and using blackout curtains to block light. For those who wake between 2–4 a.m., a small snack combining protein and fat—like a turkey roll-up or 1 tablespoon of almond butter—may help stabilize overnight blood sugar and reduce further sleep disruption, particularly for individuals sensitive to glucose swings.

To manage emotional eating, consider trying a simple three-step routine that many find helpful.

- Pause: name the feeling driving the urge — stress, boredom, anxiety — then take five slow, deep breaths to trigger the parasympathetic response and create a mindful pause to assess whether your hunger is physical or emotional.

- Nourish: reach for a **protein-focused snack** that steadies blood sugar. Some options include Greek yogurt with cinnamon (*~15 g protein*), cottage cheese with berries (antioxidants + protein), hard-boiled eggs (*~6 g each*), chia pudding made with unsweetened almond milk and vanilla, or a bone-broth latte. These choices may help you feel full without a sugar spike, though individual responses can vary.

- Redirect: shift attention with a short activity — a five-minute walk, a journaling prompt such as *"What do I really need right now?"*, or ten reps of a push-pull-squat sequence to move energy and reduce tension.

Keep your kitchen stocked with **green-light comfort foods** to make better choices easier:
- roasted sweet potato wedges
- olives
- a square of 85–100% dark chocolate
- calming herbal teas (cinnamon or chamomile)
- popcorn popped at home in olive oil
- sliced apples with tahini

Rate cravings on a 0–10 scale. If the urge is above 7, drink an electrolyte beverage and wait ten minutes; if it persists, have the smallest portion that will satisfy you so you can enjoy it without overindulging.

Watch for patterns: poor sleep increases ghrelin, so after a restless night consider adding about 10–15 grams of protein at breakfast and aiming for an earlier dinner to help stabilize blood sugar and potentially reduce evening emotional eating.

RESET FOUNDATIONS

MANAGING INFLAMMATION AND CORTISOL THROUGH NUTRITION

Build each meal around 25–35 grams of protein: two large eggs **(~12g)**, 4 ounces wild salmon **(~25g)**, 4 ounces chicken breast (~35g), 1 cup Greek yogurt (~20g), or 1 cup cooked tofu (~20g). Protein supports muscle repair and stabilizes blood sugar for healthy cortisol rhythm.

Add two cups of non-starchy vegetables per meal. Leafy greens, cruciferous vegetables, and colorful peppers provide **vitamins A, C, K, minerals, and antioxidants** that may lower inflammation. The 4–8 grams of fiber per cup aids digestion and increases fullness.

Include smart carbohydrates in cupped-hand portions: 1/2 cup quinoa, oats, or beans, or a small sweet potato. These complex carbs release energy steadily, reducing blood sugar spikes that raise cortisol while providing B vitamins and fiber.

Add anti-inflammatory fats: 1–2 tablespoons olive oil, half an avocado, a handful of nuts, or 1–2 tablespoons seeds. These supply essential fatty acids for brain health and inflammation control. Olive oil offers monounsaturated fats and polyphenols with anti-inflammatory effects.

Boost anti-inflammatory potential with 1/2 cup berries, citrus fruits, and fresh herbs like basil or parsley. Use 1 teaspoon turmeric with black pepper for curcumin absorption, plus ginger and cinnamon for blood sugar regulation.

Prioritize **omega-3s** with fatty fish 2–3 times weekly (4-ounce servings). Include polyphenol sources: green tea, dark chocolate (70% cacao), and berries for antioxidant protection.

Start days with 16–24 ounces water and continue sipping throughout. Taper fluids two hours before bedtime to avoid sleep disruptions.

Maintain consistent meal timing—three meals daily plus optional protein snack. On high-stress days, eat within **60–90 minutes** of waking and pair carbohydrates with protein and fat.

Focus on whole, minimally processed foods: organic produce, whole grains, and lean proteins. Limit alcohol to 3–4 drinks weekly and avoid charred meats.

Support gut health by rotating foods for variety and including fermented foods like sauerkraut and kimchi for probiotics. Target 25–35 grams fiber daily from vegetables, legumes, chia, and flax seeds.

Eat cruciferous vegetables for liver detox support. Fresh herbs and green tea provide antioxidants that may reduce inflammation. Ensure 0.8 grams protein per kilogram body weight for liver function.

Add movement breaks:

5–10 minute post-meal walks, strength training 2–3 times weekly with compound movements, and 1–2 zone-2 cardio sessions. Avoid high-intensity workouts late at night.

CHOOSING BETWEEN STANDARD, LOW-FODMAP, GENTLE

The anti-inflammatory cortisol reset diet requires a strategic approach. Choose one of three templates: Standard, Low-FODMAP, or Gentle. Follow your chosen template for 2-4 weeks before reassessing results.

Standard	Low-FODMAP	Gentle
Ideal for women with mild bloating and stable digestion. Use a balanced plate approach: protein (25-35g per meal), non-starchy vegetables (at least half your plate), complex carbs (cupped hand size), and healthy fats (1-2 tablespoons olive oil). Limit added sugars, alcohol, and ultra-processed foods.	For IBS-like symptoms: daily bloating, gas, cramping. Replace high-FODMAP foods with alternatives (green parts of scallions instead of onions, rice instead of wheat). Reduce legumes and high-fructose fruits. After 2-4 weeks, gradually	For high sensitivity, flare-ups, or beginners. Focus on easily digestible foods: soups, stews, smoothies. Use lightly cooked vegetables, gentle carbs (rice, oats, ripe bananas), and moderate fats.

Implementation
Maintain consistency with: 25-35g protein per meal, two cups varied vegetables, carbs paired with protein and healthy fats. Select 10 "safe" meals and prepare in advance. Dedicate one day weekly to batch cooking.

Monitoring
Keep a detailed log for 10-14 days tracking: bloating, stool quality, energy, sleep, mood, waist measurements, cravings, and menstrual changes.
If symptoms improve by 70%, continue the plan. If limited improvement, consider switching from Standard to Gentle for flare-ups, or Gentle to Standard when symptoms stabilize.

Warning signs: unintentional weight loss, blood in stool, severe abdominal pain, persistent diarrhea or constipation require immediate medical consultatio

LIFESTYLE HABITS THAT CALM CORTISOL

SLEEP RITUALS THAT ACTUALLY WORK

A cortisol-calming bedtime routine can greatly improve sleep, stress, and overall health—especially for women over 40. **Start 60–90 minutes before bed to help body and mind unwind.**

- **Set the mood:** Dim lights to support melatonin and switch to warm bulbs or dimmers. Reduce screen time; if devices are unavoidable, use blue-light filters or glasses. Instead of scrolling, try light tidying, journaling, or writing a simple plan for tomorrow.

- **Food & drink:** Finish your last meal 2–3 hours before bed—think salmon, broccoli, and sweet potato to balance blood sugar. About an hour before sleep, a calming drink of water with magnesium glycinate and sea salt may help, and tart cherry juice offers natural melatonin.

- **Body relaxation:** A warm shower or Epsom salt bath eases tension and signals rest. Keep the bedroom cool (65–68°F).

- **Wind-down routine:**

5 minutes of gentle stretching or legs-up-the-wall pose
Breathing (4-7-8 technique or humming cycles)
3 minutes of brain-dumping worries onto paper

- **Consistency:** Stick to a set bedtime and wake time within 30 minutes daily. Aim for 7.5–9 hours of sleep. Get 5–10 minutes of morning sunlight to reset circadian rhythm.

- **Sleep environment:** Keep the bedroom dark, cool, and uncluttered. Use blackout curtains, eye masks, or white noise. If you can't sleep after 20 minutes, read something dull in low light until drowsy.

- **Lifestyle tweaks:** Limit alcohol (avoid 3–4 hours before bed), stop caffeine by noon, hydrate during the day, and taper fluids at night. If you wake often at 2–3 a.m., try a small protein snack before bed.

Mindset: Practice slow nasal breathing and keep a short gratitude list to ease perimenopausal anxiety and shift focus away from stress.

Evening Sleep Ritual Checklist

DO	DON'T
• Dim the lights 60–90 minutes before bed	• Use bright lights in the evening
• Stop screens (or use blue-light filters)	• Scroll social media or watch TV in bed
• Journal, tidy lightly, or plan tomorrow	• Eat heavy meals right before sleep
• Finish dinner 2–3 hours before bed	• Drink alcohol within 3–4 hours of bedtime
• Try a calming drink (magnesium + water, or tart cherry juice)	• Have caffeine after noon
• Take a warm shower or Epsom salt bath	• Overhydrate late in the evening
• Do 5 minutes of gentle stretching or legs-up-the-wall	• Stay in bed awake for more than 20 minutes
• Practice 4-7-8 breathing or humming cycles	
• Write down worries ("brain dump")	
• Keep bedroom cool (65–68°F), dark, and uncluttered	
• Get 5–10 minutes of natural light in the morning	
• Track sleep patterns for 1 week and adjust gradually	
• Note gratitude before sleep	

GENTLE MOVEMENT VS. EXHAUSTIVE WORKOUTS

For women over 40, shifting from intense workouts to moderate, cortisol-aware movement can better support health and well-being. While some thrive on high intensity, many benefit from syncing exercise with the body's rhythms. The sweet spot is 20–30 minutes of low-to-moderate activity that energizes instead of draining, improving both physical fitness and mental balance.

Walking is one of the simplest forms of gentle movement. Aim for nasal breathing to calm the nervous system and keep a "conversation pace," which means you can talk comfortably while walking. If using a tracker, target 60–70% of your maximum heart rate to support cardiovascular health without excessive cortisol spikes.

Mobility flows or yoga add flexibility and stress relief through controlled movement and deep breathwork. A simple sun salutation sequence makes a strong morning routine, improving circulation and focus. Move slowly, letting inhales and exhales guide transitions.

Pilates offers benefits for core strength and posture with controlled, precise movements. Exercises like the hundred, roll-up, and leg circles build abdominal strength, support the spine, and improve balance when performed with mindful breathing.

For **resistance work**, choose light kettlebells or resistance bands. Focus on slow tempo and proper form over speed or heavy loads. Light kettlebell swings build hip stability and core control, while resistance bands work well for steady curls or lateral raises.

Always end sessions with a **2–3 minute cooldown**. Practice nasal breathing with longer exhales to trigger the parasympathetic nervous system and add stretches for shoulders, neck, and lower back to release tension.

High-intensity or heavy lifting should be limited to **1–2 short sessions weekly** (15–25 minutes). Allow 48 hours of recovery between sessions and attempt them only after quality sleep and good energy levels. Women over 40 can be more sensitive to cortisol fluctuations, so recovery becomes critical.

QUICK & EASY ANTI-INFLAMMATORY RECIPES

ENERGIZING 10-MINUTE BREAKFASTS

1. Turmeric Chia Pudding with Berries

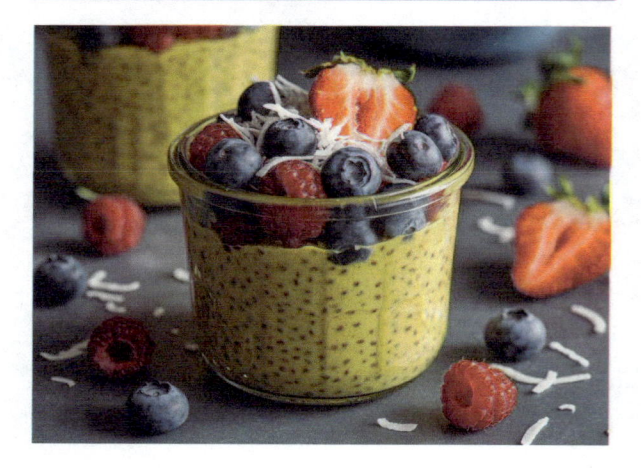

servings: 2

Ingredients

- 1 cup (240 ml) unsweetened almond milk
- 3 tablespoons (36 g) chia seeds
- 1 tablespoon (15 ml) pure maple syrup
- 1/2 teaspoon (1 g) ground turmeric
- 1/4 teaspoon (0.5 g) ground cinnamon
- 1/8 teaspoon (0.5 g) ground black pepper
- 1/2 teaspoon (2.5 ml) pure vanilla extract
- 1 cup (140 g) mixed fresh berries (blueberries, raspberries, strawberries)
- 1 tablespoon (10 g) unsweetened shredded coconut (optional)
- Pinch of sea salt

Directions

1. Add almond milk, chia seeds, maple syrup, turmeric, cinnamon, black pepper, vanilla extract, and sea salt to a medium bowl or mason jar
2. Whisk or shake vigorously for 30–60 seconds to combine and prevent clumping
3. Let sit for 2 minutes, then whisk or shake again to evenly distribute chia seeds
4. Cover and refrigerate for at least 4 hours, preferably overnight, until thickened
5. Before serving, stir well and divide between two bowls or jars
6. Top each serving with 1/2 cup (70 g) mixed berries and 1/2 tablespoon (5 g) shredded coconut if using

Estimated total time

Time: 5 min prep · 4–8 hrs chill (overnight best)

Optional swaps

Use coconut milk or oat milk for a creamier or nut-free version
Replace maple syrup with monk fruit or stevia for lower sugar
Use low-FODMAP berries (strawberries, blueberries) if needed

Nutritional facts per serving

Calories: 170
Protein: 4 g
Fat: 7 g
Carbs: 25 g
Fiber: 9 g
Sugar: 10 g

Dietary labels/tags

Gluten-free
dairy-free
vegan-friendly
low-FODMAP (with swaps)
gentle-digestion

Suggested cooking method/program

No-cook, overnight refrigerator

Storage & meal prep tips

Store covered in the refrigerator for up to 4 days
Stir before serving; add berries and coconut just before eating
Not recommended for freezing

Cortisol reset tip

Turmeric and chia seeds help lower inflammation and support steady energy, while the fiber-rich pudding keeps blood sugar balanced for a calmer morning

Possible variations

Add 1 tablespoon (16 g) almond butter for extra creaminess and healthy fats
Swap berries for diced kiwi, mango, or pomegranate seeds
Stir in 1 tablespoon (10 g) hemp seeds for more protein
For a chocolate version, add 1 teaspoon (2 g) raw cacao powder

2. Green Protein Smoothie with Spinach & Avocado

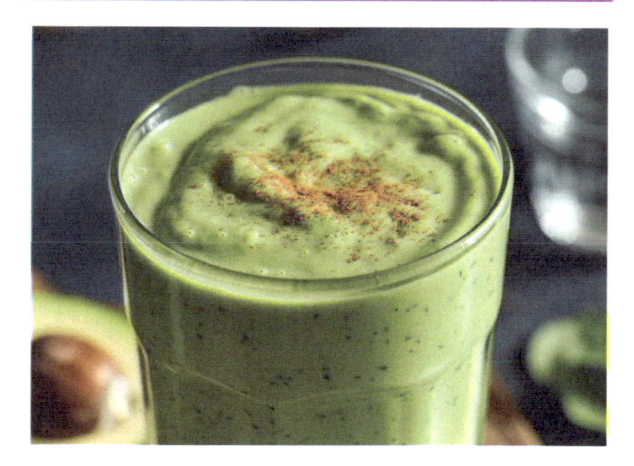

Servings: 2

Ingredients

- 2 cups (60 g) fresh baby spinach, packed
- 1 small ripe avocado (about 120 g), peeled and pitted
- 1 medium frozen banana (120 g), sliced
- 1 cup (240 ml) unsweetened almond milk
- 1/2 cup (120 ml) cold water
- 1 scoop (30 g) plant-based protein powder (unflavored or vanilla)
- 1 tablespoon (10 g) ground flaxseed
- 1 tablespoon (15 ml) fresh lemon juice
- 1/2 teaspoon (2.5 ml) pure vanilla extract
- 1/4 teaspoon (1 g) ground cinnamon
- Pinch of sea salt
- 1/2 cup (70 g) ice cubes

Directions

1. Add spinach, avocado, frozen banana, almond milk, water, protein powder, flaxseed, lemon juice, vanilla extract, cinnamon, sea salt, and ice cubes to a high-speed blender
2. Blend on high for 45–60 seconds until completely smooth and creamy
3. Taste and adjust sweetness or thickness by adding more banana or a splash of almond milk as needed
4. Pour into two glasses and serve immediately

Estimated total time

Prep time: 5 minutes
Total: 5 minutes

Optional swaps

Use coconut milk or oat milk for a creamier or nut-free version
Replace banana with 1/2 cup (75 g) frozen mango for a lower-sugar option
Choose a low-FODMAP protein powder if needed

Nutritional facts per serving

Calories: 210
Protein: 13 g
Fat: 10 g
Carbs: 20 g
Fiber: 7 g
Sugar: 6 g

Dietary labels/tags

Gluten-free
dairy-free
vegan-friendly
low-FODMAP (with swaps)
gentle-digestion

Suggested cooking method/program

No-cook, high-speed blender

Storage & meal prep tips

Best enjoyed immediately for maximum freshness
If needed, store in a sealed jar in the refrigerator for up to 24 hours; shake well before drinking
Not recommended for freezing

Cortisol reset tip

Spinach and avocado provide magnesium and healthy fats to support adrenal health, while plant protein and fiber help stabilize blood sugar and reduce stress-driven cravings

Possible variations

Add 1 tablespoon (16 g) almond butter for extra creaminess and healthy fats
Swap spinach for baby kale or a mix of greens
Stir in 1 teaspoon (2 g) spirulina or matcha for an extra antioxidant boost. Top with hemp seeds or pumpkin seeds for crunch and added minerals

3. Smoked Salmon Avocado Rye Toast

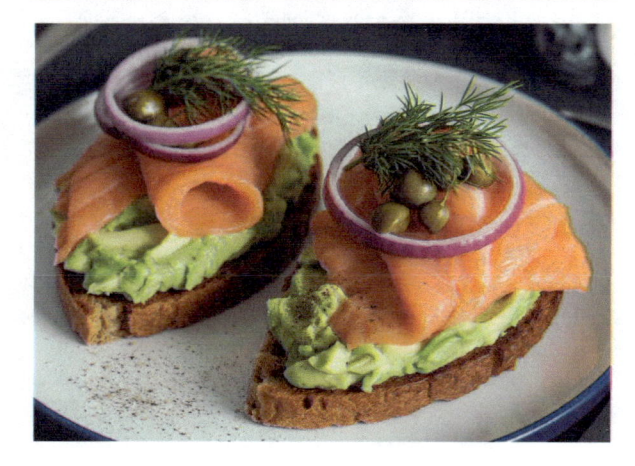

servings: 2

Ingredients

- 2 slices (60 g) sprouted rye bread
- 1 ripe avocado (about 120 g), peeled and pitted
- 1 teaspoon (5 ml) fresh lemon juice
- 1/8 teaspoon (0.5 g) sea salt
- 1/8 teaspoon (0.5 g) ground black pepper
- 3 ounces (85 g) wild-caught smoked salmon
- 1/4 small red onion (15 g), thinly sliced
- 1 tablespoon (4 g) fresh dill, chopped
- 1 teaspoon (5 g) capers, drained (optional)

Directions

1. Toast rye bread slices in a toaster or toaster oven until golden and crisp
2. In a small bowl, mash avocado with lemon juice, sea salt, and black pepper until mostly smooth
3. Spread mashed avocado evenly over each slice of toasted bread
4. Layer smoked salmon evenly on top of the avocado
5. Top with red onion slices, sprinkle with fresh dill, and add capers if using
6. Serve immediately

Estimated total time

Prep time: 5 minutes
Total: 5 minutes

Optional swaps

Use gluten-free bread for a gluten-free version
Replace rye with 100% whole grain or low-FODMAP bread if needed
Omit onion and capers for low-FODMAP

Nutritional facts per serving

Calories: 240
Protein: 13 g
Fat: 13 g
Carbs: 20 g
Fiber: 6 g
Sugar: 2 g

Dietary labels/tags

Gluten-free (with swap)
dairy-free
pescatarian
low-FODMAP (with swaps)
gentle-digestion

Suggested cooking method/program

No-cook, toaster

Storage & meal prep tips

Best enjoyed immediately for optimal texture
If prepping ahead, store mashed avocado in an airtight container with extra lemon juice to prevent browning; assemble just before eating.
Not recommended for freezing

Cortisol reset tip

Wild-caught salmon provides anti-inflammatory omega-3s to help regulate cortisol, while avocado's healthy fats and fiber support steady energy and satiety

Possible variations

Add sliced cucumber or radish for extra crunch
Swap dill for chives or parsley
Top with a sprinkle of hemp seeds for added protein and minerals
Use smoked trout or mackerel instead of salmon for variety

4. Microwave Flaxseed Oat Bowl with Blueberries

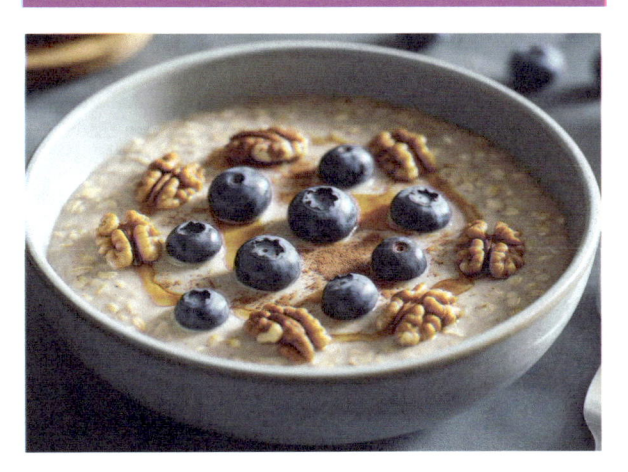

Servings: 1

Ingredients

- 1/2 cup (45 g) old-fashioned rolled oats (gluten-free if needed)
- 1 tablespoon (10 g) ground flaxseed
- 1/2 cup (120 ml) unsweetened almond milk
- 1/2 cup (120 ml) water
- 1/2 cup (75 g) fresh or frozen blueberries
- 1/2 teaspoon (2.5 ml) pure vanilla extract
- 1/4 teaspoon (1 g) ground cinnamon
- Pinch of sea salt
- 1 teaspoon (7 g) raw honey or pure maple syrup (optional)
- 1 tablespoon (10 g) chopped walnuts or pecans (optional)

Directions

1. In a microwave-safe bowl (at least 2-cup/500 ml capacity), combine oats, ground flaxseed, almond milk, water, blueberries, vanilla extract, cinnamon, and sea salt
2. Stir well to mix
3. Microwave on high for 2 minutes
4. Carefully remove (bowl will be hot) and stir again
5. If desired, drizzle with honey or maple syrup and sprinkle with chopped nuts
6. Serve warm

Estimated total time

Prep time: 3 minutes
Cook time: 2 minutes
Total: 5 minutes

Optional swaps

Use certified gluten-free oats for gluten-free
Swap almond milk for oat, coconut, or dairy milk
Replace blueberries with raspberries or diced apple
Omit nuts for nut-free

Nutritional facts per serving

Calories: 230
Protein: 6 g
Fat: 7 g
Carbs: 36 g
Fiber: 7 g
Sugar: 7 g

Dietary labels/tags

Gluten-free (with swap)
dairy-free
vegan-friendly (with maple syrup)
low-FODMAP (with swaps)
gentle-digestion

Suggested cooking method/program

Microwave, single bowl

Storage & meal prep tips

Best enjoyed immediately
To prep ahead, combine dry ingredients in a jar; add liquids and microwave when ready
Not recommended for freezing

Cortisol reset tip

Flaxseed and oats provide fiber and lignans to support hormone balance, while blueberries deliver antioxidants to help lower inflammation and support steady energy

Possible variations

Add 1 tablespoon (16 g) almond butter for extra creaminess
Top with chia seeds or hemp hearts for added protein
Stir in 1/4 cup (60 g) unsweetened applesauce for natural sweetness. Use sliced banana or strawberries instead of blueberries for variety

5. Cinnamon Walnut Quinoa Breakfast Bowl

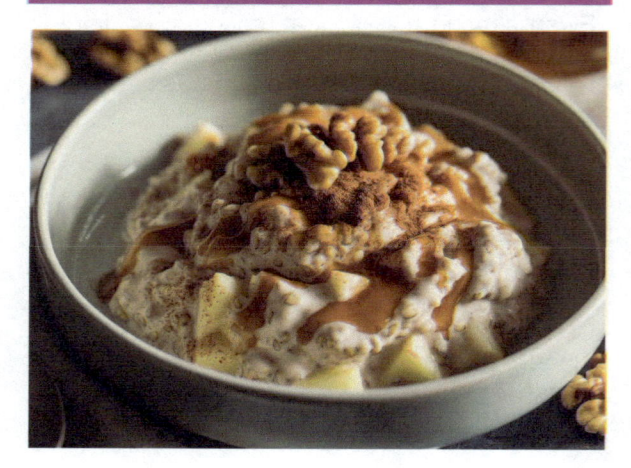

servings: 1

Ingredients

- 1/2 cup (85 g) cooked quinoa (prepared in advance or use quick-cook)
- 1/4 cup (60 ml) unsweetened almond milk
- 1/2 small apple (60 g), diced
- 1 tablespoon (7 g) chopped walnuts
- 1 tablespoon (10 g) ground flaxseed
- 1/2 teaspoon (1 g) ground cinnamon
- 1 teaspoon (7 g) raw honey or pure maple syrup (optional)
- Pinch of sea salt

Directions

1. In a small saucepan, combine cooked quinoa, almond milk, diced apple, ground cinnamon, and sea salt
2. Warm over medium heat for 3–4 minutes, stirring occasionally, until heated through and apples begin to soften
3. Stir in ground flaxseed and half the chopped walnuts
4. Transfer to a serving bowl
5. Drizzle with honey or maple syrup if using
6. Top with remaining walnuts
7. Serve warm

Estimated total time

Prep time: 3 minutes
Cook time: 7 minutes
Total: 10 minutes

Optional swaps

Use certified gluten-free quinoa for gluten-free
Swap almond milk for oat, coconut, or dairy milk
Replace apple with pear or berries
Omit walnuts for nut-free
Use pumpkin seeds or sunflower seeds instead of walnuts

Nutritional facts per serving

Calories: 260
Protein: 7 g
Fat: 11 g
Carbs: 36 g
Fiber: 6 g
Sugar: 9 g

Dietary labels/tags

Gluten-free (with swap)
dairy-free
vegan-friendly (with maple syrup)
low-FODMAP (with swaps)
gentle-digestion

Suggested cooking method/program

Stovetop, single saucepan

Storage & meal prep tips

Store cooked quinoa in an airtight container in the refrigerator for up to 4 days
Assemble bowl ingredients and reheat gently on the stovetop or in the microwave before serving
Not recommended for freezing

Cortisol reset tip

Quinoa and walnuts provide plant-based protein and magnesium to help stabilize blood sugar and support healthy cortisol rhythms, while cinnamon helps reduce inflammation and cravings

Possible variations

Add 1 tablespoon (16 g) almond butter for extra creaminess
Top with chia seeds or hemp hearts for added protein
Use sliced banana or berries instead of apple
Sprinkle with unsweetened coconut flakes for a tropical twist

LUNCH BOWLS & WRAPS

6. Ginger-Turmeric Chicken Power Bowl

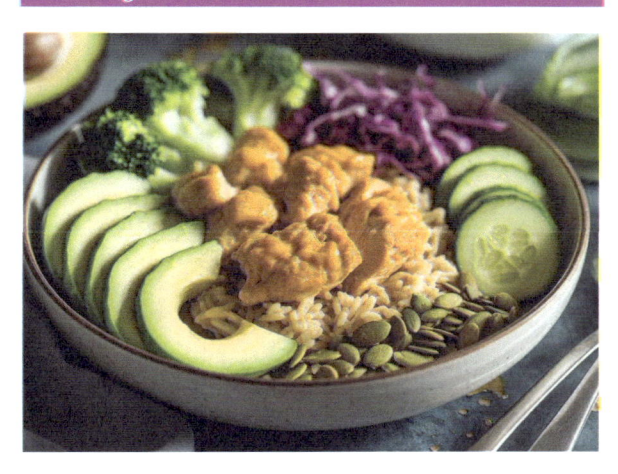

servings: 1

Ingredients

- 4 oz (115 g) boneless, skinless chicken breast, cut into bite-size pieces
- 1/2 teaspoon (2 g) ground turmeric
- 1/2 teaspoon (2 g) ground ginger or 1 teaspoon (5 g) freshly grated ginger
- 1/4 teaspoon (1 g) garlic powder
- 1 tablespoon (15 ml) extra-virgin olive oil, divided
- 1/2 cup (85 g) cooked brown rice or quinoa
- 1/2 cup (75 g) steamed broccoli florets
- 1/2 cup (50 g) shredded red cabbage
- 1/4 cup (35 g) sliced cucumber
- 1/4 avocado (35 g), sliced
- 1 tablespoon (15 ml) fresh lemon juice
- 1/8 teaspoon (0.5 g) sea salt
- 1/8 teaspoon (0.5 g) black pepper
- 1 tablespoon (10 g) pumpkin seeds (pepitas)

Directions

1. In a small bowl, toss chicken pieces with turmeric, ginger, garlic powder, 1/2 tablespoon (7 ml) olive oil, sea salt, and black pepper
2. Heat remaining 1/2 tablespoon (7 ml) olive oil in a nonstick skillet over medium-high heat
3. Add seasoned chicken and sauté for 6–8 minutes, stirring occasionally, until cooked through and golden
4. While chicken cooks, arrange cooked brown rice or quinoa in a wide bowl
5. Top with steamed broccoli, shredded red cabbage, sliced cucumber, and avocado
6. Add cooked chicken on top
7. Drizzle with fresh lemon juice
8. Sprinkle with pumpkin seeds
9. Serve immediately

Estimated total time

Prep time: 7 minutes
Cook time: 8 minutes
Total: 15 minutes

Optional swaps

Use tofu or tempeh instead of chicken for plant-based
Swap brown rice/quinoa for cauliflower rice for grain-free/low-carb
Use coconut aminos instead of salt for low-sodium
Omit pumpkin seeds for nut/seed-free
Use kale or spinach instead of cabbage

Nutritional facts per serving

Calories: 410
Protein: 29 g
Fat: 20 g
Carbs: 32 g
Fiber: 8 g
Sugar: 3 g

Dietary labels/tags

Gluten-free
dairy-free
anti-inflammatory
high-protein
gentle-digestion

Suggested cooking method/program

One-pan skillet

Storage & meal prep tips

Store assembled bowls (without avocado and lemon juice) in airtight containers in the refrigerator for up to 3 days
Add fresh avocado and lemon juice just before serving
Reheat chicken and rice/quinoa gently in the microwave or on the stovetop

Cortisol reset tip

Ginger and turmeric are powerful anti-inflammatory spices that help regulate cortisol and support immune health, while avocado and pumpkin seeds provide healthy fats for steady energy

Possible variations

Add a handful of baby spinach or arugula for extra greens
Top with a dollop of plain Greek yogurt (dairy or non-dairy) for creaminess
Swap broccoli for roasted sweet potato cubes
Use grilled salmon or shrimp instead of chicken for variety

7. Lemon-Tahini Salmon Grain Bowl

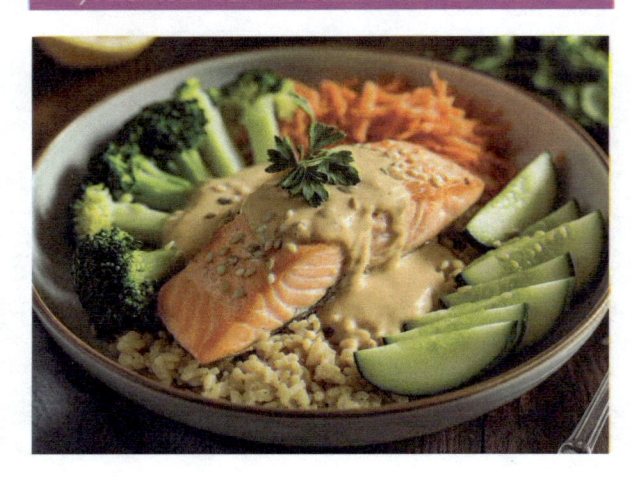

servings: 1

Ingredients

- 4 oz (115 g) wild-caught salmon fillet, skin removed
- 1/2 cup (85 g) cooked brown rice or quinoa
- 1/2 cup (75 g) steamed broccoli florets
- 1/2 cup (50 g) shredded carrots
- 1/4 cup (35 g) sliced cucumber
- 1 tablespoon (15 ml) tahini
- 1 tablespoon (15 ml) fresh lemon juice
- 1 teaspoon (5 ml) extra-virgin olive oil
- 1/8 teaspoon (0.5 g) sea salt
- 1/8 teaspoon (0.5 g) black pepper
- 1 tablespoon (10 g) hemp seeds
- 1 tablespoon (4 g) chopped fresh parsley

Directions

1. Pat salmon dry and season both sides with sea salt and black pepper
2. Heat olive oil in a nonstick skillet over medium-high heat
3. Add salmon and cook for 3–4 minutes per side, until golden and cooked through
4. In a small bowl, whisk together tahini and lemon juice with 1 tablespoon (15 ml) water until smooth and pourable
5. Arrange cooked brown rice or quinoa in a wide bowl
6. Top with steamed broccoli, shredded carrots, and sliced cucumber
7. Place cooked salmon on top of the vegetables
8. Drizzle with lemon-tahini sauce
9. Sprinkle with hemp seeds and chopped parsley
10. Serve immediately

Estimated total time

Prep time: 7 minutes
Cook time: 8 minutes
Total: 15 minutes

Optional swaps

Use certified gluten-free grains for gluten-free
Swap brown rice/quinoa for cauliflower rice for grain-free/low-carb
Use sunflower seed butter instead of tahini for nut/seed allergies
Replace salmon with tofu or tempeh for plant-based

Nutritional facts per serving

Calories: 420
Protein: 28 g
Fat: 20 g
Carbs: 34 g
Fiber: 7 g
Sugar: 4 g

Dietary labels/tags

Gluten-free (with swap)
dairy-free
anti-inflammatory
high-protein
gentle-digestion

Suggested cooking method/program

One-pan skillet

Storage & meal prep tips

Store assembled bowls (without sauce) in airtight containers in the refrigerator for up to 2 days
Add lemon-tahini sauce just before serving
Reheat salmon and grains gently in the microwave or on the stovetop

Cortisol reset tip

Wild salmon provides omega-3s to reduce inflammation and support hormone balance, while tahini and hemp seeds offer magnesium for stress resilience

Possible variations

Add a handful of baby spinach or arugula for extra greens
Top with sliced avocado for more healthy fats
Swap broccoli for roasted zucchini or asparagus - Use grilled shrimp or chicken instead of salmon for variety.

8. Warm Lentil Spinach Bowl with Walnuts

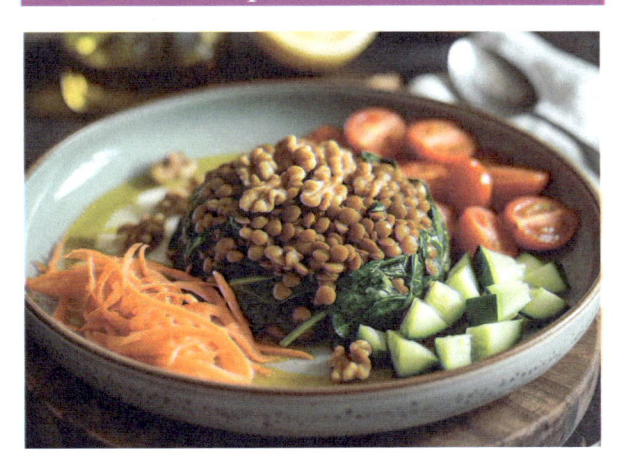

servings: 1

Ingredients

- 1/2 cup (100 g) cooked lentils (drained and rinsed if canned)
- 1 cup (30 g) baby spinach, packed
- 1/2 cup (75 g) cherry tomatoes, halved
- 1/4 cup (35 g) diced cucumber
- 1/4 cup (30 g) shredded carrots
- 1 tablespoon (7 g) chopped walnuts
- 1 tablespoon (15 ml) extra-virgin olive oil
- 1 tablespoon (15 ml) fresh lemon juice
- 1/8 teaspoon (0.5 g) sea salt
- 1/8 teaspoon (0.5 g) black pepper
- 1/4 teaspoon (1 g) ground cumin
- 1/4 teaspoon (1 g) smoked paprika

Directions

1. In a small skillet, heat olive oil over medium heat
2. Add cooked lentils, cumin, smoked paprika, sea salt, and black pepper
3. Sauté for 2–3 minutes, stirring, until lentils are warmed and fragrant
4. Add baby spinach to the skillet and cook for 1–2 minutes, stirring, until just wilted
5. Remove from heat
6. In a wide bowl, arrange shredded carrots, cherry tomatoes, and diced cucumber
7. Spoon the warm lentil-spinach mixture over the vegetables
8. Drizzle with fresh lemon juice
9. Sprinkle with chopped walnuts
10. Serve immediately

Estimated total time

Prep time: 5 minutes
Cook time: 10 minutes
Total: 15 minutes

Optional swaps

Use pecans or pumpkin seeds instead of walnuts for nut-free
Swap lentils for chickpeas or white beans
Use arugula or kale instead of spinach
Omit tomatoes for low-FODMAP

Nutritional facts per serving

Calories: 340
Protein: 13 g
Fat: 19 g
Carbs: 32 g
Fiber: 10 g
Sugar: 5 g

Dietary labels/tags

Gluten-free
dairy-free
vegan-friendly
anti-inflammatory
gentle-digestion

Suggested cooking method/program

One-pan skillet

Storage & meal prep tips

Store assembled bowls (without walnuts and lemon juice) in airtight containers in the refrigerator for up to 3 days
Add walnuts and lemon juice just before serving
Reheat lentil-spinach mixture gently in the microwave or on the stovetop

Cortisol reset tip

Lentils provide plant-based protein and fiber for steady blood sugar, while walnuts offer omega-3s and magnesium to help calm stress hormones

Possible variations

Add sliced avocado for extra healthy fats
Top with a spoonful of plain Greek yogurt (dairy or non-dairy) for creaminess
Swap carrots for roasted sweet potato cubes.
Add a sprinkle of hemp or chia seeds for more texture and nutrients

9. Mediterranean Chickpea & Kale Wrap

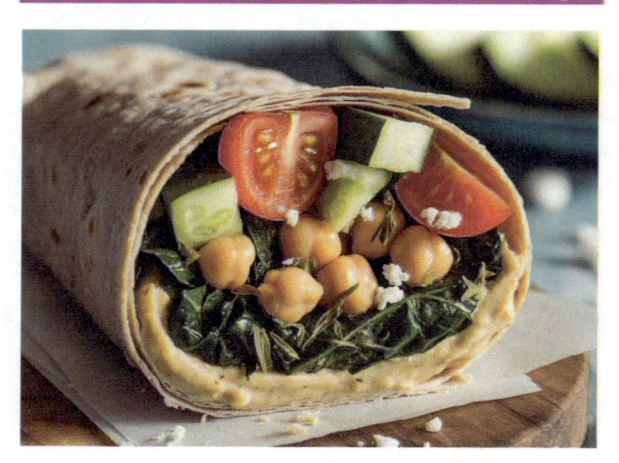

servings: 1

Ingredients

- 1/2 cup (85 g) canned chickpeas, drained and rinsed
- 1 cup (30 g) chopped kale, stems removed
- 1/4 cup (35 g) diced cucumber
- 1/4 cup (40 g) cherry tomatoes, quartered
- 2 tablespoons (30 g) hummus
- 1 tablespoon (15 ml) extra-virgin olive oil
- 1 tablespoon (15 ml) fresh lemon juice
- 1/8 teaspoon (0.5 g) sea salt
- 1/8 teaspoon (0.5 g) black pepper
- 1/4 teaspoon (1 g) dried oregano
- 1 large (50 g) gluten-free or whole grain wrap
- 1 tablespoon (10 g) crumbled feta cheese (optional)

Directions

1. In a medium skillet, heat olive oil over medium heat
2. Add chopped kale and sauté for 2–3 minutes, stirring, until just wilted
3. Add chickpeas, sea salt, black pepper, and dried oregano
4. Cook for 2–3 minutes, stirring, until chickpeas are warmed through
5. Remove from heat and drizzle with fresh lemon juice
6. Lay the wrap flat on a clean surface
7. Spread hummus evenly over the center of the wrap
8. Layer sautéed kale and chickpeas, then top with diced cucumber and cherry tomatoes
9. Sprinkle with crumbled feta cheese if using
10. Fold in the sides and roll up tightly to form a wrap
11. Slice in half and serve immediately

Estimated total time

Prep time: 7 minutes
Cook time: 8 minutes
Total: 15 minutes

Optional swaps

Use a certified gluten-free wrap for gluten-free
Omit feta for dairy-free/vegan
Swap kale for baby spinach or arugula
Use tahini instead of hummus for a different flavor

Nutritional facts per serving

Calories: 370
Protein: 12 g
Fat: 17 g
Carbs: 44 g
Fiber: 9 g
Sugar: 5 g

Dietary labels/tags

Gluten-free (with swap)
dairy-free (with swap)
vegan-friendly (with swap)
anti-inflammatory
gentle-digestion

Suggested cooking method/program

One-pan skillet

Storage & meal prep tips

Wraps can be assembled (without tomatoes and cucumber) and stored in an airtight container in the refrigerator for up to 2 days
Add fresh vegetables just before serving for best texture

Reheat the chickpea-kale mixture separately if desired

Cortisol reset tip

Chickpeas and kale provide plant-based protein, fiber, and magnesium to help stabilize blood sugar and support adrenal health, while olive oil and oregano offer anti-inflammatory benefits

Possible variations

Add sliced avocado for extra healthy fats
Swap hummus for baba ganoush or white bean spread
Include roasted red peppers or artichoke hearts for more Mediterranean flavor. Use collard greens or large lettuce leaves instead of a wrap for a grain-free option

10. Avocado Hummus Veggie Wrap

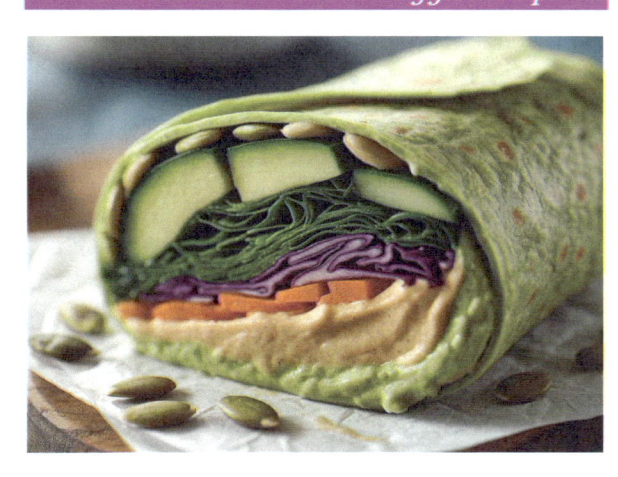

servings: 1

Ingredients

- 1 large (50 g) gluten-free or whole grain wrap
- 1/2 medium (70 g) ripe avocado
- 1/4 cup (60 g) hummus
- 1/2 cup (35 g) baby spinach, packed
- 1/4 cup (30 g) shredded purple cabbage
- 1/4 cup (35 g) grated carrot
- 1/4 cup (35 g) sliced cucumber
- 1 tablespoon (15 ml) fresh lemon juice
- 1/8 teaspoon (0.5 g) sea salt
- 1/8 teaspoon (0.5 g) black pepper
- 1 tablespoon (10 g) pumpkin seeds (optional)

Directions

1. In a small bowl, mash avocado with lemon juice, sea salt, and black pepper until mostly smooth
2. Lay the wrap flat on a clean surface
3. Spread hummus evenly over the center of the wrap
4. Layer mashed avocado, baby spinach, shredded cabbage, grated carrot, and sliced cucumber
5. Sprinkle with pumpkin seeds if using
6. Fold in the sides and roll up tightly to form a wrap
7. Slice in half and serve immediately, or wrap tightly in parchment for on-the-go

Estimated total time

Prep time: 7 minutes
Cook time: 3 minutes
Total: 10 minutes

Optional swaps

Use a certified gluten-free wrap for gluten-free
Swap hummus for white bean dip or baba ganoush
Omit pumpkin seeds for nut/seed-free
Use arugula or kale instead of spinach
For low-FODMAP, use a low-FODMAP hummus and limit avocado to 1/8 fruit

Nutritional facts per serving

Calories: 360
Protein: 9 g
Fat: 20 g
Carbs: 39 g
Fiber: 10 g
Sugar: 5 g

Dietary labels/tags

Gluten-free (with swap)
Dairy-free
Vegan-friendly
Anti-inflammatory
Gentle-digestion

Suggested cooking method/program

No-cook, quick assembly

Storage & meal prep tips

Wraps can be assembled (without avocado) and stored in an airtight container in the refrigerator for up to 1 day

Add mashed avocado just before serving to prevent browning
Wrap tightly in parchment or foil for easy transport

Cortisol reset tip

Avocado and pumpkin seeds provide magnesium and healthy fats to help regulate stress hormones, while colorful veggies offer antioxidants to reduce inflammation

Possible variations

Add sliced roasted red peppers or artichoke hearts for extra flavor
Swap spinach for mixed greens or romaine
Include a sprinkle of hemp seeds or chia seeds for more texture
Add a few fresh basil or cilantro leaves for a herby twist

ONE-PAN 20-MINUTE DINNERS (5 RECIPES)

11. Lemon-Garlic Turmeric Shrimp Skillet

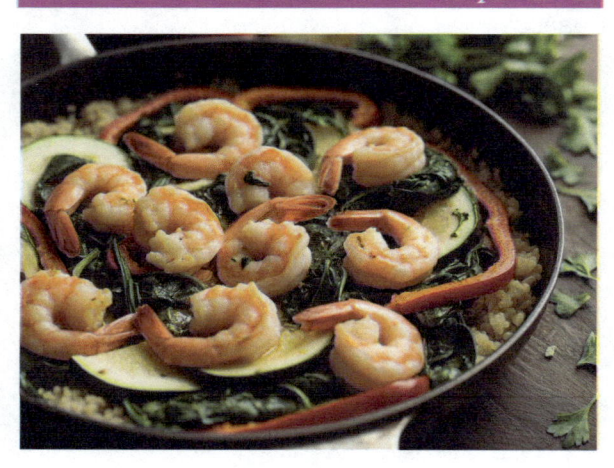

servings: 2

Ingredients

- 12 ounces (340 g) large raw shrimp, peeled and deveined
- 1 tablespoon (15 ml) extra-virgin olive oil
- 1/2 medium (60 g) red bell pepper, thinly sliced
- 1/2 medium (60 g) zucchini, halved and sliced
- 1 cup (30 g) baby spinach, packed
- 2 cloves garlic, minced
- 1/2 teaspoon (1 g) ground turmeric
- 1/4 teaspoon (0.5 g) smoked paprika
- 1/4 teaspoon (0.5 g) sea salt
- 1/8 teaspoon (0.5 g) black pepper
- 2 tablespoons (30 ml) fresh lemon juice
- 1 teaspoon (2 g) lemon zest
- 2 tablespoons (8 g) chopped fresh parsley
- 1/2 cup (90 g) cooked quinoa or brown rice (optional, for serving)

Directions

1. Pat shrimp dry with paper towels and season with turmeric, smoked paprika, sea salt, and black pepper
2. Heat olive oil in a large nonstick skillet over medium heat
3. Add minced garlic and sauté for 30 seconds until fragrant
4. Add red bell pepper and zucchini; cook for 3–4 minutes, stirring occasionally, until just tender
5. Push vegetables to the side of the skillet and add shrimp in a single layer
6. Cook shrimp for 2–3 minutes per side, or until pink and opaque
7. Add baby spinach and toss everything together; cook for 1 minute until spinach wilts
8. Drizzle with fresh lemon juice and sprinkle with lemon zest
9. Remove from heat and garnish with chopped parsley
10. Serve immediately over cooked quinoa, brown rice, or cauliflower rice if desired

Estimated total time

Prep time: 7 minutes
Cook time: 13 minutes
Total: 20 minutes

Optional swaps

Use cauliflower rice for grain-free/low-carb
Omit quinoa/rice for paleo
Swap zucchini for yellow squash or asparagus
Use ghee instead of olive oil for dairy flavor

Nutritional facts per serving

Calories: 260 (without quinoa/rice)
Protein: 28 g
Fat: 10 g
Carbs: 11 g
Fiber: 3 g
Sugar: 4 g

Dietary labels/tags

Gluten-free

Dairy-free
Paleo-friendly (with swap)
Anti-inflammatory
Gentle-digestion

Suggested cooking method/program

One-pan skillet

Storage & meal prep tips

Store leftovers in an airtight container in the refrigerator for up to 2 days
Reheat gently in a skillet over low heat to avoid overcooking shrimp
Best enjoyed fresh for optimal texture

Cortisol reset tip

Turmeric and lemon provide anti-inflammatory support, while shrimp offers lean protein to help stabilize blood sugar and support adrenal health

Possible variations

Add a pinch of red pepper flakes for heat
Include sliced mushrooms or snap peas for extra veggies. Swap shrimp for wild-caught salmon chunks or chicken breast strips. Top with toasted pumpkin seeds for crunch and added magnesium.

12. Dijon Salmon with Asparagus & Sunflower Seeds

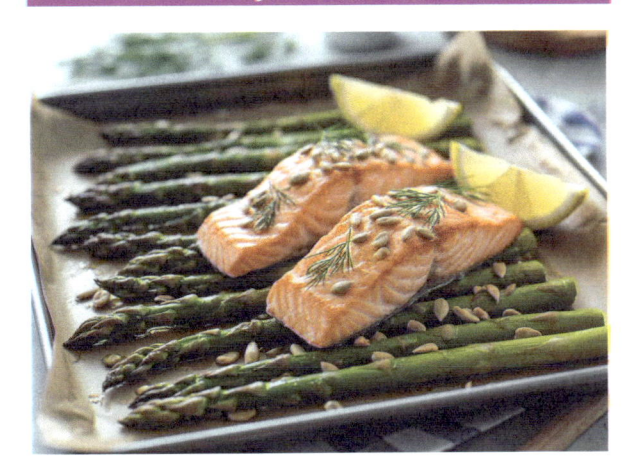

servings: 2

Ingredients

- 2 wild-caught salmon fillets (5 oz/140 g each)
- 1 tablespoon (15 g) Dijon mustard
- 1 tablespoon (15 ml) extra-virgin olive oil
- 1 teaspoon (5 ml) pure maple syrup
- 1/2 teaspoon (1 g) garlic powder
- 1/4 teaspoon (0.5 g) sea salt
- 1/4 teaspoon (0.5 g) black pepper
- 8 ounces (225 g) fresh asparagus, trimmed
- 1 tablespoon (10 g) raw sunflower seeds
- 1 tablespoon (4 g) chopped fresh dill or parsley
- Lemon wedges, for serving

Directions

1. Preheat oven to 400°F (200°C). Line a large rimmed baking sheet with parchment paper.
2. In a small bowl, whisk together Dijon mustard, olive oil, maple syrup, garlic powder, sea salt, and black pepper.
3. Pat salmon fillets dry with paper towels. Place them skin-side down on one side of the prepared baking sheet.
4. Brush the Dijon mixture evenly over the tops of the salmon fillets.
5. Arrange asparagus spears on the other side of the baking sheet. Drizzle with a little extra olive oil and sprinkle with a pinch of salt and pepper. Toss to coat and spread in a single layer.
6. Roast in the oven for 12–15 minutes, until salmon is just cooked through and flakes easily with a fork, and asparagus is crisp-tender.
7. Remove from oven. Sprinkle sunflower seeds and fresh dill or parsley over the asparagus.
8. Serve salmon and asparagus immediately with lemon wedges on the side.

Estimated total time

Prep time: 5 minutes
Cook time: 15 minutes
Total: 20 minutes

Optional swaps

Use whole grain mustard instead of Dijon
Swap maple syrup for raw honey
For low-FODMAP, omit garlic powder and use garlic-infused olive oil
Use pumpkin seeds instead of sunflower seeds for nut/seed preference
Substitute asparagus with broccolini or green beans

Nutritional facts per serving

Calories: 340

Protein: 29 g
Fat: 20 g
Carbs: 10 g
Fiber: 3 g
Sugar: 4 g

Dietary labels/tags

Gluten-free
Dairy-free
Paleo-friendly (with swap)
Anti-inflammatory
Gentle-digestion

Suggested cooking method/program

One-pan oven roast

Storage & meal prep tips

Store leftovers in an airtight container in the refrigerator for up to 2 days
Reheat gently in a 300°F oven or enjoy cold over salad greens
Best texture when enjoyed fresh

Cortisol reset tip

Wild salmon provides omega-3s to help lower inflammation and support hormone balance, while sunflower seeds add magnesium for stress resilience

Possible variations

Add sliced cherry tomatoes to the pan for extra color
Top salmon with a sprinkle of hemp seeds for more healthy fats
Swap dill for basil or cilantro for a different flavor profile
Serve over a bed of cooked quinoa or cauliflower rice for a heartier meal

13. Coconut-Ginger Tofu & Broccoli Stir-Skillet

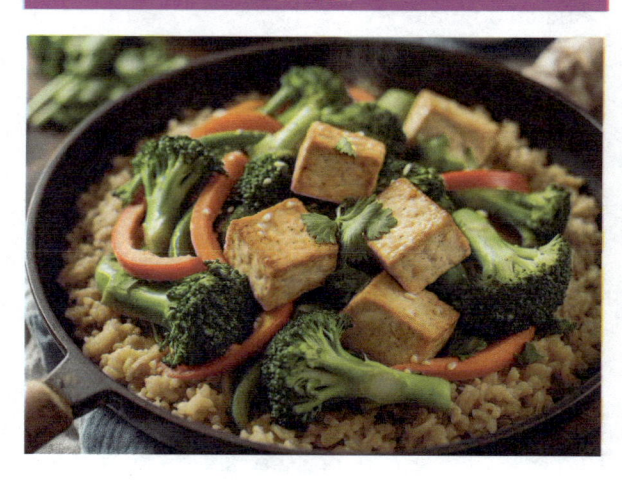

servings: 2

Ingredients

- 14 ounces (400 g) extra-firm tofu, drained and pressed
- 1 tablespoon (15 ml) avocado oil or coconut oil
- 2 cups (140 g) broccoli florets
- 1/2 medium (60 g) red bell pepper, thinly sliced
- 1/2 cup (80 g) thinly sliced carrots
- 2 cloves garlic, minced
- 1 tablespoon (10 g) fresh ginger, grated
- 1/2 cup (120 ml) light coconut milk (canned, shaken)
- 1 tablespoon (15 ml) coconut aminos or low-sodium tamari
- 1 teaspoon (5 ml) toasted sesame oil
- 1/4 teaspoon (0.5 g) sea salt
- 1/8 teaspoon (0.5 g) black pepper
- 2 tablespoons (8 g) chopped fresh cilantro or basil
- 1 teaspoon (2 g) sesame seeds, for garnish
- 1/2 cup (90 g) cooked brown rice or cauliflower rice (optional, for serving)

Directions

1. Cut tofu into 3/4-inch cubes and pat dry with paper towels
2. Heat avocado oil in a large nonstick skillet over medium-high heat
3. Add tofu cubes in a single layer; cook for 4–5 minutes, turning occasionally, until golden on most sides

4. Push tofu to the side of the skillet; add broccoli, red bell pepper, and carrots
5. Sauté vegetables for 3–4 minutes, stirring occasionally, until just tender
6. Add minced garlic and grated ginger; cook for 1 minute until fragrant
7. Pour in coconut milk and coconut aminos; stir to combine
8. Season with sea salt and black pepper
9. Simmer for 2–3 minutes, stirring gently, until sauce thickens slightly and vegetables are crisp-tender
10. Drizzle with toasted sesame oil and toss everything together
11. Remove from heat; sprinkle with chopped cilantro or basil and sesame seeds
12. Serve immediately over cooked brown rice or cauliflower rice if desired

Estimated total time

Prep time: 7 minutes
Cook time: 13 minutes
Total: 20 minutes

Optional swaps

Use tamari for gluten-free
Swap coconut aminos for soy-free
Use snap peas or green beans instead of broccoli
Replace tofu with tempeh or cooked chicken breast for non-vegan

Nutritional facts per serving

Calories: 320 (without rice)
Protein: 18 g
Fat: 20 g
Carbs: 17 g
Fiber: 5 g
Sugar: 5 g

Dietary labels/tags

Gluten-free (with tamari)
Dairy-free
Vegan-friendly
Anti-inflammatory
Gentle-digestion

Suggested cooking method/program

One-pan skillet

Storage & meal prep tips

Store leftovers in an airtight container in the refrigerator for up to 3 days
Reheat gently in a skillet over low heat, adding a splash of coconut milk if needed
Best enjoyed within 2 days for optimal texture

Cortisol reset tip

Ginger and coconut milk offer anti-inflammatory benefits, while tofu provides plant-based protein to help stabilize blood sugar and support hormone balance

Possible variations

Add a pinch of red pepper flakes for gentle heat
Top with chopped cashews or pumpkin seeds for crunch
Swap cilantro for mint or parsley Stir in a handful of baby spinach at the end for extra greens

14. Herbed Chicken Thighs with Zucchini and Olives

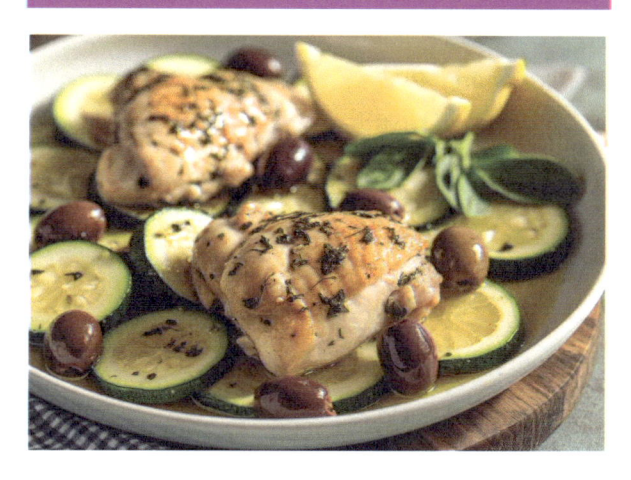

servings: 2

Ingredients

- 4 boneless, skinless chicken thighs (about 16 oz / 450 g)
- 1 tablespoon (15 ml) extra-virgin olive oil
- 1/2 teaspoon (1 g) sea salt
- 1/4 teaspoon (0.5 g) black pepper
- 1 teaspoon (2 g) dried Italian herb blend (or 1/2 teaspoon each dried oregano and thyme)
- 2 medium zucchini (about 12 oz / 340 g), sliced into 1/2-inch rounds
- 1/2 cup (75 g) pitted Kalamata olives, halved
- 2 cloves garlic, minced
- 1 tablespoon (4 g) chopped fresh parsley or basil

- 1 tablespoon (15 ml) fresh lemon juice
- Lemon wedges, for serving

Directions

1. Pat chicken thighs dry with paper towels. Season both sides with sea salt, black pepper, and Italian herb blend.
2. Heat olive oil in a large nonstick skillet over medium-high heat.
3. Add chicken thighs in a single layer. Sear for 3–4 minutes per side, until golden brown.
4. Push chicken to the side of the skillet. Add zucchini rounds and olives to the pan. Sauté for 3–4 minutes, stirring occasionally, until zucchini is just tender.
5. Add minced garlic to the pan. Cook for 1 minute, stirring, until fragrant.
6. Drizzle lemon juice over chicken and vegetables. Toss gently to combine and cook for 1–2 more minutes, until chicken is cooked through (internal temperature 165°F) and zucchini is crisp-tender.
7. Remove from heat. Sprinkle with chopped parsley or basil.
8. Serve immediately with lemon wedges on the side.

Estimated total time

Prep time: 5 minutes
Cook time: 15 minutes
Total: 20 minutes

Optional swaps

Use boneless, skinless chicken breast for lower fat
Swap Italian herb blend for herbes de Provence
For low-FODMAP, omit garlic and use garlic-infused olive oil
Use green olives instead of Kalamata
Replace zucchini with yellow squash or eggplant

Nutritional facts per serving

Calories: 340
Protein: 32 g
Fat: 18 g
Carbs: 9 g
Fiber: 3 g
Sugar: 4 g

Dietary labels/tags

Gluten-free
Dairy-free
Paleo-friendly
Anti-inflammatory
Gentle-digestion

Storage & meal prep tips

Store leftovers in an airtight container in the refrigerator for up to 3 days
Reheat gently in a skillet over low heat or in the microwave until warmed through
Best texture when enjoyed fresh

Cortisol reset tip

Chicken thighs provide steady protein to help stabilize blood sugar, while olives and olive oil offer healthy fats and polyphenols to reduce inflammation and support hormone balance

Possible variations

Add a handful of cherry tomatoes to the pan for extra color and antioxidants
Top with toasted pine nuts for crunch
Swap parsley for fresh dill or mint. Serve over cooked quinoa or cauliflower rice for a more filling meal.

15. Sweet Potato, Kale & Lentil Hash with Tahini Drizzle

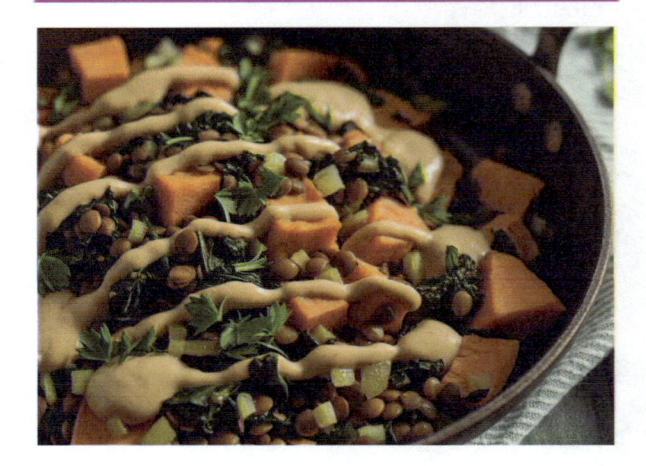

servings: 2

Ingredients

- 1 medium (8 oz / 225 g) sweet potato, peeled and diced into 1/2-inch cubes
- 1 tablespoon (15 ml) avocado oil
- 1/2 cup (80 g) yellow onion, finely diced
- 2 cloves garlic, minced
- 1 teaspoon (2 g) ground cumin

- 1/2 teaspoon (1 g) smoked paprika
- 1/4 teaspoon (0.5 g) sea salt
- 1/8 teaspoon (0.5 g) black pepper
- 1 cup (150 g) cooked brown or green lentils, drained and rinsed
- 2 cups (60 g) chopped kale, stems removed
- 2 tablespoons (30 ml) water
- 2 tablespoons (30 g) tahini
- 1 tablespoon (15 ml) fresh lemon juice
- 1 teaspoon (5 ml) maple syrup
- 1 tablespoon (15 ml) warm water (for tahini sauce)
- 1 tablespoon (4 g) chopped fresh parsley, for garnish

Directions

1. Heat avocado oil in a large nonstick skillet over medium heat
2. Add diced sweet potato and onion; sauté for 5–6 minutes, stirring occasionally, until sweet potato begins to soften
3. Stir in minced garlic, ground cumin, smoked paprika, sea salt, and black pepper; cook for 1 minute until fragrant
4. Add cooked lentils and chopped kale to the skillet
5. Pour in 2 tablespoons water, cover, and steam for 3–4 minutes until kale is wilted and sweet potato is fork-tender
6. Uncover and cook for 1–2 more minutes, stirring gently, until any excess moisture evaporates
7. In a small bowl, whisk together tahini, lemon juice, maple syrup, and 1 tablespoon warm water until smooth and pourable
8. Drizzle tahini sauce over the hash in the skillet
9. Sprinkle with chopped parsley and serve immediately

Estimated total time

Prep time: 7 minutes
Cook time: 13 minutes
Total: 20 minutes

Optional swaps

Use baby spinach instead of kale
Swap sweet potato for butternut squash
For low-FODMAP, omit garlic and onion and use garlic-infused oil
Use canned lentils for convenience

Nutritional facts per serving

Calories: 340
Protein: 13 g
Fat: 14 g
Carbs: 46 g
Fiber: 10 g
Sugar: 9 g

Dietary labels/tags

Gluten-free
Dairy-free
Vegan-friendly
Anti-inflammatory
Gentle-digestion

Suggested cooking method/program

One-pan skillet

Storage & meal prep tips

Store leftovers in an airtight container in the refrigerator for up to 3 days
Reheat gently in a skillet over low heat, adding a splash of water if needed
Tahini drizzle can be stored separately and added just before serving

Cortisol reset tip

Sweet potatoes and lentils provide steady complex carbs and fiber to help balance blood sugar, while tahini and kale offer magnesium and antioxidants to support stress resilience

Possible variations

Top with a fried or poached egg for extra protein
Add a pinch of chili flakes for gentle heat
Swap parsley for fresh cilantro or dill
Stir in diced red bell pepper for more color and vitamin C

NO-BAKE SNACKS & SWEET FIXES

16. Turmeric Almond Energy Bites

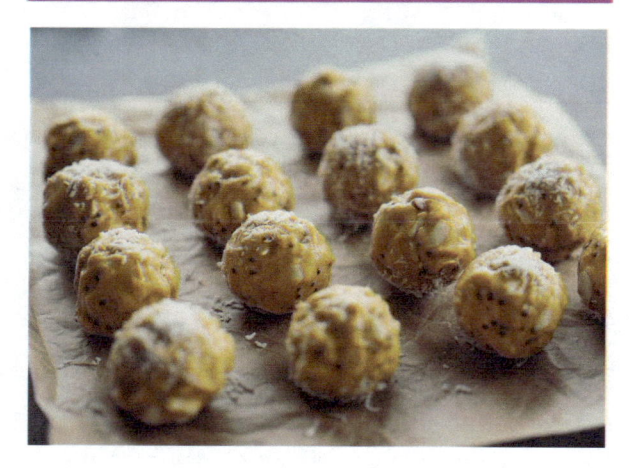

servings: 8 (2 bites per serving)

Ingredients

- 1 cup (140 g) raw almonds
- 1/2 cup (80 g) Medjool dates, pitted (about 6 large)
- 2 tablespoons (16 g) ground flaxseed
- 1 tablespoon (7 g) chia seeds
- 1 tablespoon (15 ml) almond butter
- 1 tablespoon (15 ml) pure maple syrup
- 1 teaspoon (2 g) ground turmeric
- 1/4 teaspoon (0.5 g) ground cinnamon
- 1/8 teaspoon (0.25 g) fine sea salt
- 1/2 teaspoon (2 ml) pure vanilla extract
- 1–2 teaspoons (5–10 ml) water, as needed
- 2 tablespoons (12 g) unsweetened shredded coconut, for rolling (optional)

Directions

1. Add raw almonds to a food processor. Pulse 8–10 times until coarsely chopped.
2. Add pitted dates, ground flaxseed, chia seeds, almond butter, maple syrup, ground turmeric, cinnamon, sea salt, and vanilla extract.
3. Process for 30–45 seconds, scraping down sides as needed, until mixture is finely chopped and sticky.
4. If mixture is too dry to hold together, add water 1 teaspoon at a time and pulse until it forms a dough that holds when pressed.
5. Scoop out 1 tablespoon (about 20 g) of mixture and roll tightly into a ball. Repeat to make 16 bites.
6. Roll each bite in shredded coconut, if using, to coat.
7. Place bites on a parchment-lined plate. Refrigerate for at least 20 minutes to firm up before serving.

Estimated total time

Prep time: 10 minutes
Cook time: 0 minutes
Total: 10 minutes

Optional swaps

Use cashews or walnuts instead of almonds
Swap almond butter for sunflower seed butter (nut-free)
For low-FODMAP, use maple syrup only and limit to 1 bite per serving
Omit shredded coconut for coconut-free

Nutritional facts per serving

Calories: 180
Protein: 4 g
Fat: 11 g
Carbs: 18 g
Fiber: 4 g
Sugar: 10 g

Dietary labels/tags

Gluten-free
Dairy-free
Vegan-friendly
Anti-inflammatory
No added refined sugar
Gentle-digestion

Suggested cooking method/program

No-bake, food processor

Storage & meal prep tips

Store in an airtight container in the refrigerator for up to 1 week
Freeze for up to 2 months; thaw at room temperature for 10 minutes before eating
Great for grab-and-go snacks or lunchboxes

Cortisol reset tip

Turmeric and almonds provide anti-inflammatory compounds and healthy fats to help stabilize blood sugar and support hormone balance, while dates offer natural sweetness without spiking cortisol.

Possible variations

Add 2 tablespoons mini dark chocolate chips for a treat
Mix in 1 tablespoon hemp seeds for extra omega-3s
Swap cinnamon for ground ginger for a different flavor
Roll in finely chopped pistachios instead of coconut

17. Ginger-Date Walnut Bars

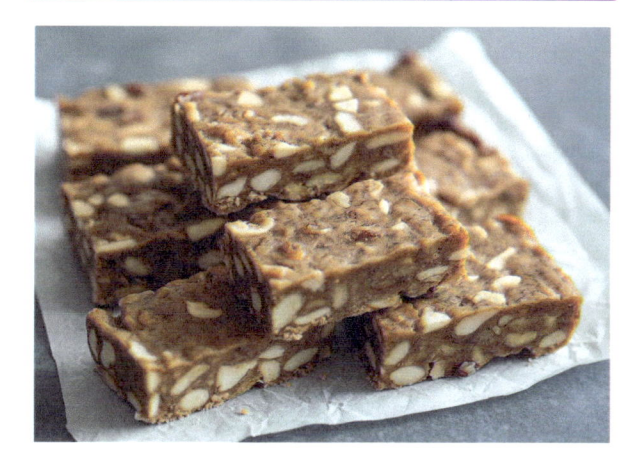

servings: 8 (1 bar per serving)

Ingredients

- 1 cup (120 g) raw walnuts
- 1/2 cup (80 g) Medjool dates, pitted (about 6 large)
- 1/4 cup (20 g) unsweetened shredded coconut
- 2 tablespoons (16 g) ground flaxseed
- 1 tablespoon (15 ml) pure maple syrup
- 1 tablespoon (6 g) finely chopped crystallized ginger
- 1 teaspoon (2 g) ground ginger
- 1/4 teaspoon (0.5 g) fine sea salt
- 1/2 teaspoon (2 ml) pure vanilla extract
- 1–2 teaspoons (5–10 ml) water, as needed

Directions

1. Add raw walnuts to a food processor. Pulse 8–10 times until coarsely chopped.
2. Add pitted dates, shredded coconut, ground flaxseed, maple syrup, crystallized ginger, ground ginger, sea salt, and vanilla extract.
3. Process for 30–45 seconds, scraping down sides as needed, until mixture is finely chopped and sticky.
4. If mixture is too dry to hold together, add water 1 teaspoon at a time and pulse until it forms a dough that holds when pressed.
5. Line a 9 x 5-inch loaf pan with parchment paper, leaving overhang for easy removal.
6. Transfer mixture to the pan and press firmly and evenly into a compact layer using a spatula or the back of a measuring cup.
7. Refrigerate for at least 20 minutes to firm up.
8. Lift out of the pan and slice into 8 bars.

Estimated total time

Prep time: 10 minutes
Cook time: 0 minutes
Total: 10 minutes

Optional swaps

Use pecans or almonds instead of walnuts
Swap crystallized ginger for 1 tablespoon (6 g) chopped dried apricots for less spice
For low-FODMAP, use maple syrup only and limit to 1/2 bar per serving
Omit coconut for coconut-free

Nutritional facts per serving

Calories: 170
Protein: 3 g
Fat: 12 g
Carbs: 15 g
Fiber: 3 g
Sugar: 9 g

Dietary labels/tags

Gluten-free
Dairy-free
Vegan-friendly
Anti-inflammatory
No added refined sugar
Gentle-digestion

Suggested cooking method/program

No-bake, food processor

Storage & meal prep tips

Store bars in an airtight container in the refrigerator for up to 1 week
Freeze for up to 2 months; thaw at room temperature for 10 minutes before eating
Great for lunchboxes or afternoon snacks

Cortisol reset tip

Walnuts and flaxseed provide omega-3s and fiber to help reduce inflammation and support hormone balance, while ginger offers natural anti-inflammatory benefits for stress resilience.

Possible variations

Add 2 tablespoons mini dark chocolate chips for a treat
Mix in 1 tablespoon chia seeds for extra fiber
Swap vanilla for almond extract for a different flavor
Top with a sprinkle of hemp seeds before pressing into the pan

18. Berry-Chia Lemon Cups

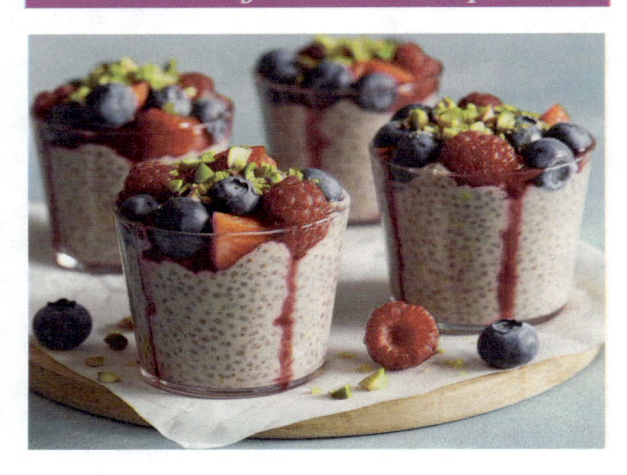

servings: 6 (1 cup per serving)

Ingredients

- 1 cup (150 g) fresh mixed berries (blueberries, raspberries, strawberries, chopped)
- 1 cup (240 ml) unsweetened almond milk
- 1/4 cup (40 g) chia seeds
- 2 tablespoons (30 ml) pure maple syrup
- 1 tablespoon (6 g) finely grated lemon zest
- 2 tablespoons (30 ml) fresh lemon juice
- 1/2 teaspoon (2 ml) pure vanilla extract
- Pinch fine sea salt
- 1/4 cup (30 g) unsalted raw pistachios, chopped (optional, for topping)

Directions

1. In a medium mixing bowl, whisk together almond milk, chia seeds, maple syrup, lemon zest, lemon juice, vanilla extract, and sea salt until well combined.
2. Let the mixture sit for 5 minutes, then whisk again to prevent clumping.
3. Gently fold in the mixed berries.
4. Divide the mixture evenly among 6 small cups or jars (about 1/3 cup per serving).
5. Cover and refrigerate for at least 20 minutes, or until thickened to a pudding-like consistency.
6. Before serving, top each cup with chopped pistachios, if using.

Estimated total time

Prep time: 10 minutes
Cook time: 0 minutes
Total: 10 minutes

Optional swaps

Use coconut milk or oat milk instead of almond milk
Swap maple syrup for raw honey (not vegan)
For low-FODMAP, use only blueberries and limit to 1/2 cup berries per serving
Omit pistachios for nut-free

Nutritional facts per serving

Calories: 120
Protein: 3 g
Fat: 5 g
Carbs: 17 g
Fiber: 6 g
Sugar: 8 g

Dietary labels/tags

Gluten-free
Dairy-free
Vegan-friendly
Anti-inflammatory
No added refined sugar
Gentle-digestion

Suggested cooking method/program

No-bake, refrigerator set

Storage & meal prep tips

Store covered in the refrigerator for up to 4 days. Best enjoyed chilled; do not freeze as texture may change
Great for breakfast, snack, or dessert

Cortisol reset tip

Chia seeds and berries provide fiber and antioxidants to help regulate blood sugar and reduce inflammation, while lemon supports gentle detoxification and adrenal health.

Possible variations

Add 1/2 teaspoon ground ginger for a zesty kick
Top with unsweetened coconut flakes instead of pistachios
Use all blueberries for a milder flavor

19. Coconut Matcha Yogurt Parfaits

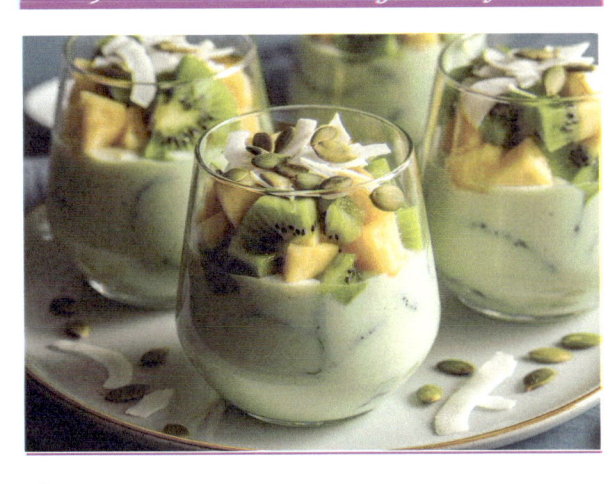

servings: 4 (about 1 cup per serving)

Ingredients

- 2 cups (480 g) unsweetened coconut yogurt
- 2 teaspoons (4 g) ceremonial-grade matcha powder
- 2 tablespoons (30 ml) pure maple syrup
- 1 teaspoon (5 ml) pure vanilla extract
- 1 cup (150 g) fresh kiwi, peeled and diced
- 1 cup (150 g) fresh pineapple, diced
- 1/2 cup (40 g) unsweetened coconut flakes
- 1/4 cup (30 g) raw pumpkin seeds (pepitas)
- Pinch fine sea salt

Directions

1. In a medium bowl, whisk together coconut yogurt, matcha powder, maple syrup, vanilla extract, and sea salt until smooth and evenly green
2. Layer 1/4 cup matcha yogurt mixture into the bottom of each of 4 small glasses or jars
3. Add a layer of diced kiwi and pineapple (about 1/4 cup total fruit per parfait)
4. Sprinkle 1 tablespoon coconut flakes and 1 tablespoon pumpkin seeds over the fruit layer
5. Repeat layers with remaining matcha yogurt, fruit, coconut flakes, and pumpkin seeds
6. Serve immediately, or cover and refrigerate for up to 2 hours for a chilled parfait

Estimated total time

Prep time: 10 minutes
Cook time: 0 minutes
Total: 10 minutes

Optional swaps

Use plain Greek yogurt (dairy) or almond yogurt instead of coconut yogurt
Swap maple syrup for raw honey (not vegan)
For low-FODMAP, use lactose-free yogurt and limit fruit to 1/2 cup per serving
Omit pumpkin seeds for nut-free

Nutritional facts per serving

Calories: 210
Protein: 4 g
Fat: 12 g
Carbs: 23 g
Fiber: 4 g
Sugar: 13 g

Dietary labels/tags

Gluten-free
Dairy-free
Vegan-friendly
Anti-inflammatory
No added refined sugar
Gentle-digestion

Suggested cooking method/program

No-bake, refrigerator set

Storage & meal prep tips

Store covered in the refrigerator for up to 2 days
Best enjoyed within 24 hours for optimal texture
Do not freeze; fruit may become watery

Cortisol reset tip

Matcha provides L-theanine for calm focus, while coconut yogurt and seeds offer healthy fats and probiotics to support gut and adrenal health.

Possible variations

Use mango or papaya instead of pineapple for a tropical twist

Top with hemp seeds or chopped walnuts for extra crunch
Add a layer of unsweetened granola for more texture
Swirl in 1 tablespoon almond butter for richness

ENERGIZING BREAKFASTS

SMOOTHIE & SHAKE RECIPES

20. Golden Turmeric Oat Smoothie

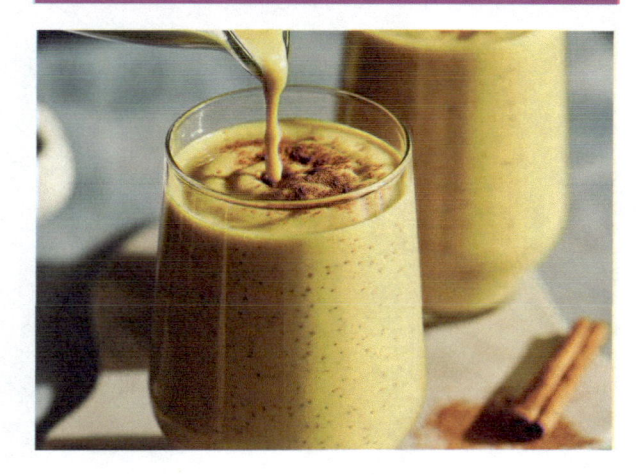

servings: 2 (about 12 oz per serving)

Ingredients

- 1 cup (240 ml) unsweetened almond milk
- 1/2 cup (45 g) gluten-free rolled oats
- 1 medium ripe banana (about 120 g), sliced and frozen
- 1/2 cup (120 g) plain coconut yogurt
- 1 tablespoon (15 ml) pure maple syrup
- 1 teaspoon (2 g) ground turmeric
- 1/2 teaspoon (1 g) ground cinnamon
- 1/4 teaspoon (1 g) ground ginger
- 1/8 teaspoon (0.5 g) fine sea salt
- 1/4 teaspoon (1 ml) pure vanilla extract
- 1 tablespoon (10 g) chia seeds
- 1/2 cup (120 ml) ice cubes
- Pinch black pepper (to enhance turmeric absorption)

Directions

1. Add almond milk, rolled oats, frozen banana, coconut yogurt, maple syrup, turmeric, cinnamon, ginger, sea salt, vanilla extract, chia seeds, ice cubes, and black pepper to a high-speed blender
2. Blend on high for 1–2 minutes until completely smooth and creamy, scraping down sides as needed
3. Taste and adjust sweetness or spice as desired
4. Pour into 2 large glasses
5. Serve immediately, garnished with a sprinkle of cinnamon or extra chia seeds if desired

Estimated total time

Prep time: 5 minutes
Cook time: 0 minutes
Total: 5 minutes

Optional swaps

Use oat milk or cashew milk instead of almond milk
Swap coconut yogurt for Greek yogurt (not dairy-free)
For low-FODMAP, use lactose-free yogurt and limit banana to 1/3 medium per serving
Omit chia seeds for seed-free

Nutritional facts per serving

Calories: 210
Protein: 5 g
Fat: 6 g
Carbs: 37 g
Fiber: 6 g
Sugar: 13 g

Dietary labels/tags

Gluten-free
Dairy-free
Vegan-friendly
Anti-inflammatory
No added refined sugar
Gentle-digestion

Suggested cooking method/program

No-cook, high-speed blender

Storage & meal prep tips

Best enjoyed immediately for optimal texture
If storing, refrigerate in a sealed jar for up to 12 hours; shake well before drinking as oats and chia may thicken the smoothie
Not recommended for freezing

Cortisol reset tip

Turmeric and ginger provide potent anti-inflammatory support, while oats and chia seeds offer steady energy and fiber to help balance blood sugar and support adrenal health.

Possible variations

Add 1 scoop plant-based vanilla protein powder for extra protein
Use 1/2 cup frozen mango instead of banana for a tropical twist
Stir in 1 tablespoon almond butter for richness
Top with toasted coconut flakes or pumpkin seeds for crunch

21. Berry Collagen Cortisol-Balance Smoothie

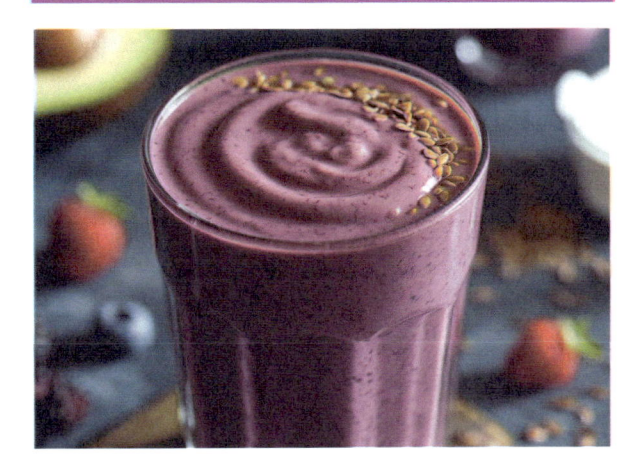

servings: 2 (about 12 oz per serving)

Ingredients

- 1 cup (150 g) frozen mixed berries (blueberries, raspberries, strawberries)
- 1 cup (240 ml) unsweetened almond milk
- 1/2 cup (120 g) plain coconut yogurt
- 1 scoop (10 g) unflavored or vanilla collagen peptides
- 1 tablespoon (15 ml) pure maple syrup
- 1 tablespoon (10 g) ground flaxseed
- 1/2 small ripe avocado (about 60 g), peeled and pitted
- 1/2 teaspoon (2 g) ground cinnamon
- 1/2 teaspoon (2.5 ml) pure vanilla extract
- 1/8 teaspoon (0.5 g) fine sea salt
- 1 cup (120 g) ice cubes

Directions

1. Add frozen berries, almond milk, coconut yogurt, collagen peptides, maple syrup, ground flaxseed, avocado, cinnamon, vanilla extract, sea salt, and ice cubes to a high-speed blender
2. Blend on high for 1–2 minutes until completely smooth and creamy, scraping down sides as needed
3. Taste and adjust sweetness or thickness by adding more maple syrup or almond milk if desired
4. Pour into 2 large glasses
5. Serve immediately, garnished with extra berries or a sprinkle of flaxseed if desired

Estimated total time

Prep time: 5 minutes
Cook time: 0 minutes
Total: 5 minutes

Optional swaps

Use oat milk or cashew milk instead of almond milk
Swap coconut yogurt for Greek yogurt (not dairy-free)
For low-FODMAP, use lactose-free yogurt and limit berries to 1/2 cup per serving
Omit collagen for vegan

Nutritional facts per serving

Calories: 190
Protein: 10 g
Fat: 8 g
Carbs: 22 g
Fiber: 6 g
Sugar: 10 g

Dietary labels/tags

Gluten-free
Dairy-free
Anti-inflammatory
No added refined sugar
Gentle-digestion

Suggested cooking method/program

No-cook, high-speed blender

Storage & meal prep tips

Best enjoyed immediately for optimal texture
If storing, refrigerate in a sealed jar for up to 12 hours; shake well before drinking as flaxseed may thicken the smoothie
Not recommended for freezing

Cortisol reset tip

Collagen peptides and flaxseed support gut and hormone health, while berries and avocado provide antioxidants and healthy fats to help reduce inflammation and stabilize energy.

Possible variations

Add 1 tablespoon almond butter for extra creaminess
Stir in 1 tablespoon chia seeds for more fiber
Use all blueberries for a brain-boosting twist.

22. Avocado Matcha Energy Shake

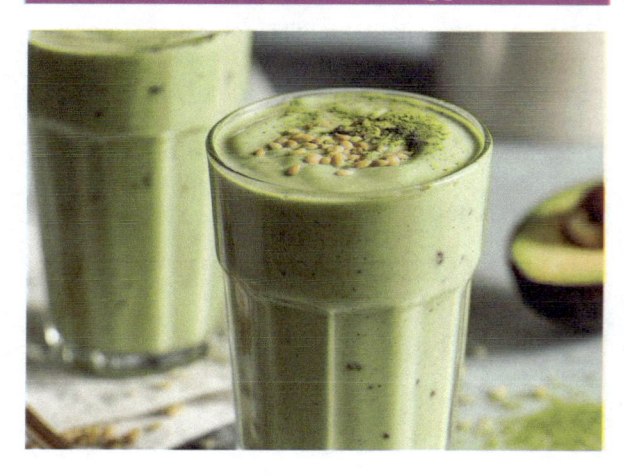

servings: 2 (about 12 oz per serving)

Ingredients

- 1 1/2 cups (360 ml) unsweetened almond milk
- 1 medium ripe avocado (about 120 g), peeled and pitted
- 1 tablespoon (6 g) ceremonial-grade matcha green tea powder
- 1/2 cup (120 g) plain coconut yogurt
- 2 tablespoons (30 ml) pure maple syrup
- 1 tablespoon (10 g) hemp seeds
- 1/2 teaspoon (2 ml) pure vanilla extract
- 1/8 teaspoon (0.5 g) fine sea salt
- 1 cup (120 g) ice cubes
- Optional: 1 scoop (10 g) unflavored or vanilla collagen peptides

Directions

1. Add almond milk, avocado, matcha powder, coconut yogurt, maple syrup, hemp seeds, vanilla extract, sea salt, ice cubes, and collagen peptides (if using) to a high-speed blender
2. Blend on high for 1–2 minutes until completely smooth and creamy, scraping down sides as needed
3. Taste and adjust sweetness or matcha intensity as desired
4. Pour into 2 large glasses
5. Serve immediately, garnished with a sprinkle of hemp seeds or a dusting of matcha if desired

Estimated total time

Prep time: 5 minutes
Cook time: 0 minutes
Total: 5 minutes

Optional swaps

Use oat milk or cashew milk instead of almond milk
Swap coconut yogurt for Greek yogurt (not dairy-free)
For low-FODMAP, use lactose-free yogurt and limit avocado to 1/8 per serving
Omit collagen for vegan

Nutritional facts per serving

Calories: 230
Protein: 6 g
Fat: 15 g
Carbs: 20 g
Fiber: 7 g
Sugar: 7 g

Dietary labels/tags

Gluten-free
Dairy-free
Vegan-friendly (if collagen omitted)
Anti-inflammatory
No added refined sugar
Gentle-digestion

Suggested cooking method/program

No-cook, high-speed blender

Storage & meal prep tips

Best enjoyed immediately for optimal texture
If storing, refrigerate in a sealed jar for up to 12 hours; shake well before drinking as the shake may thicken
Not recommended for freezing

Cortisol reset tip

Matcha provides gentle, sustained energy without the jitters, while avocado and hemp seeds deliver healthy fats and magnesium to help calm the nervous system and support hormone balance.

Possible variations

Add 1/2 frozen banana for extra creaminess and sweetness
Use 1 tablespoon almond butter for a richer texture
Stir in 1 tablespoon chia seeds for more fiber
Top with unsweetened coconut flakes or pumpkin seeds for crunch

23. Ginger Peach Protein Smoothie

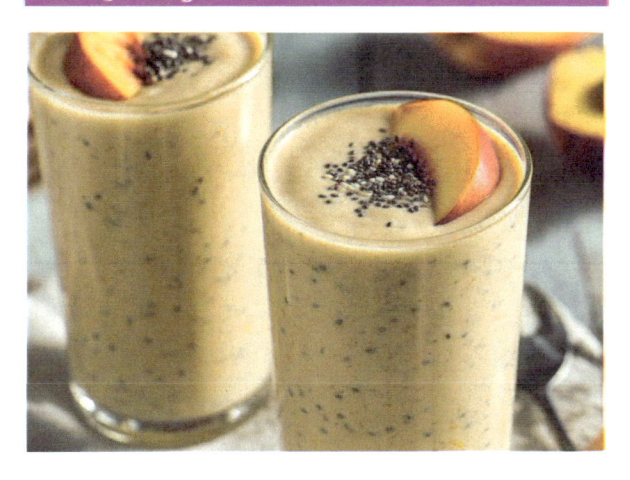

servings: 2 (about 12 oz per serving)

Ingredients

- 1 1/2 cups (225 g) frozen sliced peaches
- 1 cup (240 ml) unsweetened almond milk
- 1/2 cup (120 g) plain coconut yogurt
- 1 scoop (10 g) unflavored or vanilla plant-based protein powder
- 1 tablespoon (15 ml) pure maple syrup
- 1 tablespoon (10 g) chia seeds
- 1-inch (8 g) piece fresh ginger, peeled and grated
- 1/2 small ripe banana (about 60 g), peeled
- 1/2 teaspoon (2.5 ml) pure vanilla extract
- 1/8 teaspoon (0.5 g) fine sea salt
- 1 cup (120 g) ice cubes

Directions

1. Add frozen peaches, almond milk, coconut yogurt, protein powder, maple syrup, chia seeds, grated ginger, banana, vanilla extract, sea salt, and ice cubes to a high-speed blender
2. Blend on high for 1–2 minutes until completely smooth and creamy, scraping down sides as needed
3. Taste and adjust sweetness or ginger intensity as desired
4. Pour into 2 large glasses
5. Serve immediately, garnished with extra peach slices or a sprinkle of chia seeds if desired

Estimated total time

Prep time: 5 minutes
Cook time: 0 minutes
Total: 5 minutes

Optional swaps

Use oat milk or cashew milk instead of almond milk
Swap coconut yogurt for Greek yogurt (not dairy-free)
For low-FODMAP, use lactose-free yogurt and limit peaches to 1/2 cup per serving
Omit protein powder for a lighter smoothie

Nutritional facts per serving

Calories: 200
Protein: 11 g
Fat: 6 g
Carbs: 28 g
Fiber: 6 g
Sugar: 14 g

Dietary labels/tags

Gluten-free
Dairy-free
Vegan-friendly (if plant-based protein used)
Anti-inflammatory
No added refined sugar
Gentle-digestion

Suggested cooking method/program

No-cook, high-speed blender

Storage & meal prep tips

Best enjoyed immediately for optimal texture
If storing, refrigerate in a sealed jar for up to 12 hours; shake well before drinking as chia seeds may thicken the smoothie
Not recommended for freezing

Cortisol reset tip

Ginger and chia seeds help reduce inflammation and support digestion, while peaches and banana provide natural sweetness and steady energy to help balance cortisol levels.

Possible variations

Add 1 tablespoon almond butter for extra creaminess
Use all mango instead of peaches for a tropical twist
Stir in 1 tablespoon ground flaxseed for more fiber
Top with unsweetened coconut flakes or pumpkin seeds for crunch

24. Green Apple Spinach Detox Shake

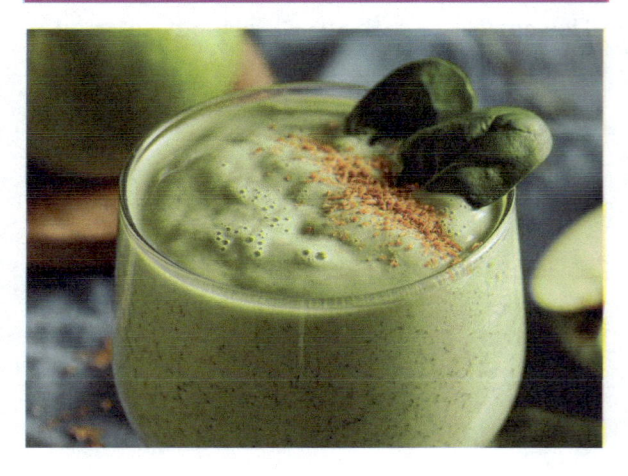

servings: 2 (about 12 oz per serving)

Ingredients

- 1 1/2 cups (225 g) chopped green apple (about 1 large, cored, skin on)
- 2 cups (60 g) baby spinach, packed
- 1 cup (240 ml) unsweetened almond milk
- 1/2 cup (120 g) plain coconut yogurt
- 1 tablespoon (15 ml) fresh lemon juice
- 1 tablespoon (10 g) ground flaxseed
- 1 tablespoon (20 g) raw honey or pure maple syrup
- 1/2 small ripe avocado (about 60 g), peeled and pitted
- 1/2 teaspoon (2.5 ml) pure vanilla extract
- 1/8 teaspoon (0.5 g) fine sea salt
- 1 cup (120 g) ice cubes
- Optional: 1 scoop (10 g) unflavored or vanilla plant-based protein powder

Directions

1. Add green apple, spinach, almond milk, coconut yogurt, lemon juice, ground flaxseed, honey or maple syrup, avocado, vanilla extract, sea salt, ice cubes, and protein powder (if using) to a high-speed blender
2. Blend on high for 1–2 minutes until completely smooth and creamy, scraping down sides as needed
3. Taste and adjust sweetness or lemon juice as desired
4. Pour into 2 large glasses
5. Serve immediately, garnished with a few spinach leaves or a sprinkle of ground flaxseed if desired

Estimated total time

Prep time: 5 minutes
Cook time: 0 minutes
Total: 5 minutes

Optional swaps

Use oat milk or cashew milk instead of almond milk
Swap coconut yogurt for Greek yogurt (not dairy-free)
For low-FODMAP, use lactose-free yogurt and limit apple to 1/2 cup per serving
Omit honey/maple syrup for a lower-sugar option
Omit protein powder for a lighter shake

Nutritional facts per serving

Calories: 190
Protein: 5 g
Fat: 8 g
Carbs: 27 g
Fiber: 7 g
Sugar: 15 g

Dietary labels/tags

Gluten-free
Dairy-free
Vegan-friendly (if plant-based protein and maple syrup used)
Anti-inflammatory
No added refined sugar
Gentle-digestion

Suggested cooking method/program

No-cook, high-speed blender

Storage & meal prep tips

Best enjoyed immediately for optimal texture
If storing, refrigerate in a sealed jar for up to 12 hours; shake well before drinking as the shake may thicken
Not recommended for freezing

Cortisol reset tip

Green apple and spinach provide vitamin C and polyphenols to help lower inflammation, while avocado and flaxseed deliver healthy fats and fiber to support steady energy and hormone balance.

Possible variations

Add 1/2 cup frozen pineapple for a tropical twist
Use kale instead of spinach for a heartier green flavor
Stir in 1 tablespoon chia seeds for extra fiber
Top with pumpkin seeds or unsweetened coconut flakes for crunch

EGG-BASED RECIPES

25. Turmeric Spinach Egg Muffins

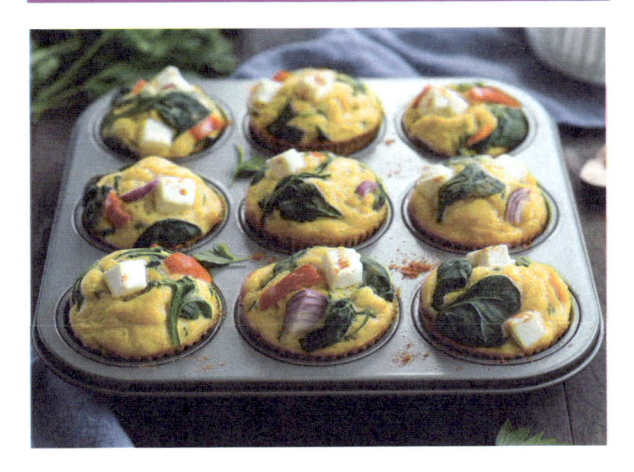

servings: 6 (2 muffins per serving)

Ingredients

- 8 large eggs
- 1/4 cup (60 ml) unsweetened almond milk
- 1 cup (30 g) baby spinach, finely chopped
- 1/2 cup (60 g) red bell pepper, finely diced
- 1/4 cup (30 g) red onion, finely diced
- 1/4 cup (30 g) crumbled feta cheese (optional, omit for dairy-free)
- 1 tablespoon (15 ml) extra-virgin olive oil
- 1 teaspoon (2 g) ground turmeric
- 1/2 teaspoon (1 g) ground black pepper
- 1/2 teaspoon (2.5 g) fine sea salt
- 1/4 teaspoon (0.5 g) smoked paprika
- Optional: 1/4 cup (10 g) fresh parsley, chopped

Directions

1. Preheat oven to 350°F (175°C). Lightly grease a 12-cup muffin tin with olive oil or line with silicone muffin liners
2. In a large mixing bowl, whisk eggs and almond milk until well combined
3. Add chopped spinach, red bell pepper, red onion, feta (if using), olive oil, turmeric, black pepper, sea salt, smoked paprika, and parsley (if using)
4. Stir mixture until vegetables and spices are evenly distributed
5. Pour egg mixture evenly into the 12 muffin cups, filling each about 3/4 full
6. Bake for 20–22 minutes, or until muffins are puffed and set in the center
7. Remove from oven and let cool in the pan for 5 minutes, then run a thin spatula around edges and transfer to a wire rack
8. Serve warm or at room temperature

Estimated total time

Prep time: 10 minutes | Cook time: 22 minutes
Total: 32 minutes

Optional swaps

Use coconut milk or oat milk instead of almond milk
Omit feta for dairy-free or swap with dairy-free cheese
For low-FODMAP, omit onion and use green tops of scallions

Nutritional facts per serving

Calories: 140
Protein: 10 g
Fat: 9 g
Carbs: 4 g
Fiber: 1 g
Sugar: 2 g

Dietary labels/tags

Gluten-free
Dairy-free option
Vegetarian
Low-carb
Anti-inflammatory
Meal-prep friendly
Gentle-digestion

Suggested cooking method/program

Oven-baked, muffin tin

Storage & meal prep tips

Cool completely before storing
Refrigerate in an airtight container up to 4 days
Reheat in microwave for 30–40 seconds or enjoy cold. Freeze up to 2 months; thaw overnight in fridge and reheat as above

Cortisol reset tip

Turmeric and spinach provide anti-inflammatory phytonutrients to help lower stress and support hormone balance, while eggs offer steady protein for all-day energy.

Possible variations

Add 1/2 cup shredded zucchini (squeeze out moisture) for extra veggies
Use kale instead of spinach
Swap red bell pepper for sun-dried tomatoes
Top with pumpkin seeds before baking for crunch and magnesium

26. Herbed Egg White Frittata with Asparagus & Sunflower Seeds

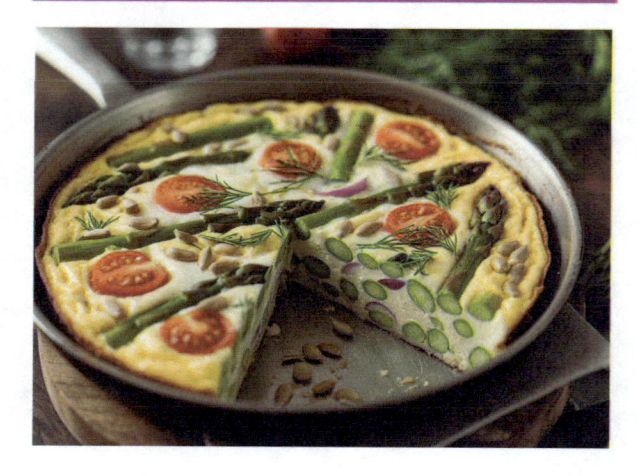

servings: 4

Ingredients

- 2 cups (480 ml) liquid egg whites or whites from 8 large eggs
- 1/4 cup (60 ml) unsweetened almond milk
- 1 cup (120 g) asparagus, trimmed and cut into 1-inch pieces
- 1/2 cup (60 g) cherry tomatoes, halved
- 1/4 cup (30 g) red onion, finely diced
- 2 tablespoons (8 g) fresh parsley, chopped
- 1 tablespoon (4 g) fresh dill, chopped
- 2 tablespoons (18 g) raw sunflower seeds
- 1 tablespoon (15 ml) extra-virgin olive oil
- 1/2 teaspoon (2.5 g) fine sea salt
- 1/4 teaspoon (0.5 g) ground black pepper
- Optional: 1/4 cup (30 g) crumbled goat cheese (omit for dairy-free)

Directions

1. Preheat oven to 375°F (190°C).
2. Heat olive oil in a 10-inch oven-safe nonstick skillet over medium heat.
3. Add asparagus and red onion; sauté for 3–4 minutes until just tender.
4. Add cherry tomatoes and cook for 1 minute more, stirring occasionally.
5. In a medium bowl, whisk together egg whites, almond milk, parsley, dill, sea salt, and black pepper until frothy.
6. Pour egg white mixture evenly over vegetables in the skillet.
7. Sprinkle sunflower seeds and goat cheese (if using) evenly over the top.
8. Cook undisturbed on the stovetop for 2–3 minutes until edges begin to set.
9. Transfer skillet to the oven and bake for 10–12 minutes, or until the center is set and the top is lightly golden.
10. Remove from oven and let cool for 5 minutes before slicing into wedges.
11. Serve warm or at room temperature.

Estimated total time

Prep time: 10 minutes
Cook time: 18 minutes
Total: 28 minutes

Optional swaps

Use oat milk or coconut milk instead of almond milk
Omit goat cheese for dairy-free
For low-FODMAP, use green tops of scallions instead of red onion and limit asparagus to 1/2 cup per serving

Nutritional facts per serving

Calories: 110
Protein: 11 g
Fat: 6 g
Carbs: 5 g
Fiber: 2 g
Sugar: 2 g

Dietary labels/tags

Gluten-free
Dairy-free option
Vegetarian
Low-carb
Anti-inflammatory
Gentle-digestion
Meal-prep friendly

Suggested cooking method/program

Oven-baked, oven-safe skillet

Storage & meal prep tips

Cool completely before storing
Refrigerate in an airtight container up to 4 days
Reheat individual slices in microwave for 30–40 seconds or enjoy cold
Not recommended for freezing due to texture changes

Cortisol reset tip

Egg whites and sunflower seeds provide lean protein and magnesium to support steady energy and hormone balance, while fresh herbs and asparagus deliver anti-inflammatory phytonutrients.

Possible variations

Add 1/2 cup (60 g) baby spinach for extra greens
Swap dill for basil or chives
Use pumpkin seeds instead of sunflower seeds
Top with sliced avocado before serving for healthy fats

27. Avocado Soft-Boiled Eggs with Lemon Zest & Hemp Seeds

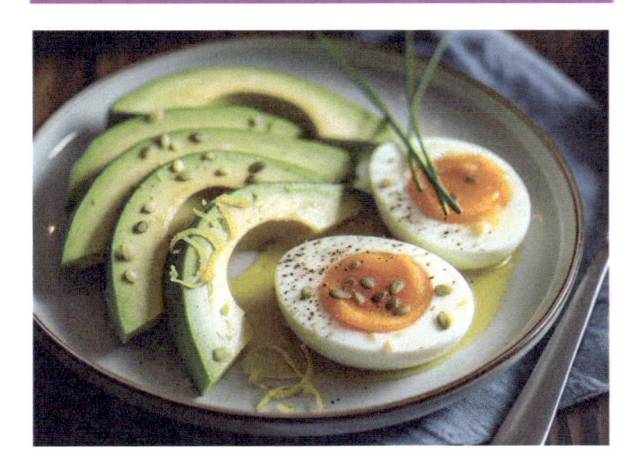

servings: 2

Ingredients

- 4 large eggs
- 1 large ripe avocado
- 1 tablespoon (15 ml) fresh lemon juice
- 1/2 teaspoon (1 g) lemon zest
- 1 tablespoon (10 g) hulled hemp seeds
- 1 tablespoon (15 ml) extra-virgin olive oil
- 1/4 teaspoon (1.5 g) fine sea salt
- 1/4 teaspoon (0.5 g) ground black pepper
- Optional: 1 tablespoon (4 g) fresh chives, finely chopped
- Optional swaps: Use lime juice and zest instead of lemon; for low-FODMAP, use only 1/4 avocado per serving

Directions

1. Bring a medium saucepan of water to a gentle boil over medium-high heat
2. Carefully lower eggs into boiling water using a spoon
3. Boil eggs for exactly 6 1/2 minutes for soft, jammy yolks
4. While eggs cook, halve avocado, remove pit, and slice each half thinly
5. When eggs are done, transfer immediately to a bowl of ice water for 2 minutes to stop cooking
6. Gently peel eggs and slice each in half lengthwise
7. Arrange avocado slices on two plates
8. Drizzle avocado with lemon juice and sprinkle with half the sea salt and black pepper
9. Place two soft-boiled egg halves on each plate beside avocado
10. Drizzle eggs and avocado with olive oil
11. Sprinkle with lemon zest, hemp seeds, remaining salt and pepper, and chives if using
12. Serve immediately

Estimated total time

Prep time: 5 minutes
Cook time: 7 minutes
Total: 12 minutes

Nutritional facts per serving

Calories: 260
Protein: 11 g
Fat: 21 g
Carbs: 7 g
Fiber: 5 g
Sugar: 1 g

Dietary labels/tags

Gluten-free
Dairy-free
Vegetarian
Low-carb
Anti-inflammatory
Gentle-digestion
Meal-prep friendly

Suggested cooking method/program

Stovetop, soft-boiled

Storage & meal prep tips

Best enjoyed fresh
If prepping ahead, store peeled eggs and sliced avocado separately in airtight containers in the fridge up to 2 days
To prevent avocado browning, brush slices with extra lemon juice and cover tightly
Not recommended for freezing

Cortisol reset tip

Avocado and hemp seeds provide magnesium and healthy fats to help regulate cortisol and support steady energy, while lemon zest adds anti-inflammatory antioxidants.

Possible variations

Top with microgreens or arugula for extra phytonutrients
Add a sprinkle of smoked paprika or chili flakes for gentle heat
Serve over a slice of gluten-free toast for a heartier meal
Swap hemp seeds for pumpkin or chia seeds for a different nutrient profile

28. Ginger-Turmeric Poached Eggs over Quinoa & Kale

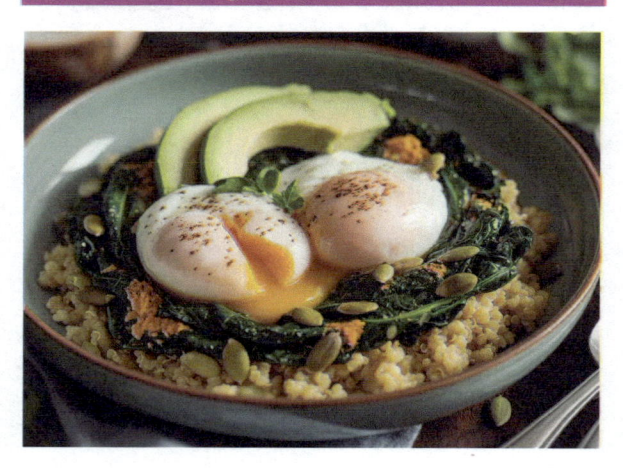

servings: 2

Ingredients

- 4 large eggs
- 1 cup (185 g) cooked quinoa
- 2 cups (60 g) baby kale, packed
- 1 tablespoon (15 ml) extra-virgin olive oil
- 1/2 teaspoon (2 g) ground turmeric
- 1/2 teaspoon (2 g) freshly grated ginger
- 1/4 teaspoon (1.5 g) fine sea salt, divided
- 1/4 teaspoon (0.5 g) ground black pepper
- 2 cups (480 ml) filtered water
- 1 tablespoon (15 ml) apple cider vinegar
- 1/2 small avocado, sliced
- 1 tablespoon (10 g) hulled pumpkin seeds
- Optional: 1 tablespoon (4 g) fresh cilantro or parsley, chopped
- Optional swaps: Use baby spinach instead of kale; for low-FODMAP, use only 1/4 avocado per serving and swap kale for baby spinach

Directions

1. Rinse and drain quinoa if uncooked; cook according to package instructions and set aside
2. In a medium skillet, heat olive oil over medium heat
3. Add grated ginger and turmeric; sauté for 1 minute until fragrant
4. Add baby kale, 1/8 teaspoon salt, and sauté for 2–3 minutes until wilted; remove from heat
5. In a medium saucepan, bring 2 cups water and apple cider vinegar to a gentle simmer (not boiling)
6. Crack each egg into a small bowl
7. Swirl simmering water with a spoon to create a gentle whirlpool
8. Carefully slide one egg at a time into the center of the whirlpool
9. Poach eggs for 3–4 minutes for soft yolks, or up to 5 minutes for firmer yolks
10. Remove eggs with a slotted spoon and drain on a paper towel
11. To assemble, divide cooked quinoa between two bowls
12. Top each with sautéed kale, two poached eggs, and avocado slices
13. Sprinkle with pumpkin seeds, remaining salt, black pepper, and fresh herbs if using
14. Serve immediately

Estimated total time

Prep time: 10 minutes
Cook time: 15 minutes
Total: 25 minutes

Nutritional facts per serving

Calories: 320
Protein: 15 g
Fat: 18 g
Carbs: 27 g
Fiber: 6 g
Sugar: 2 g

Dietary labels/tags

Gluten-free
Dairy-free
Vegetarian
Anti-inflammatory
Low-FODMAP option
Gentle-digestion
Meal-prep friendly

Suggested cooking method/program

Stovetop, poaching

Storage & meal prep tips

Store cooked quinoa and sautéed kale separately in airtight containers in the fridge up to 4 days

Poach eggs fresh for best texture; if needed, poached eggs can be made ahead and stored in cold water in the fridge for up to 2 days, then reheated in hot water for 1 minute

Avocado best sliced fresh before serving

Not recommended for freezing

Cortisol reset tip

Turmeric and ginger provide potent anti-inflammatory compounds to help regulate cortisol, while quinoa and eggs offer steady energy and support hormone balance.

Possible variations

Top with a spoonful of sauerkraut for gut health

Swap pumpkin seeds for hemp or sunflower seeds

Add a squeeze of lemon juice for brightness

Use arugula or chard instead of kale for a different green

29. Cortisol-Balancing Mediterranean Egg Bowl with Olives Tomatoes & Walnuts

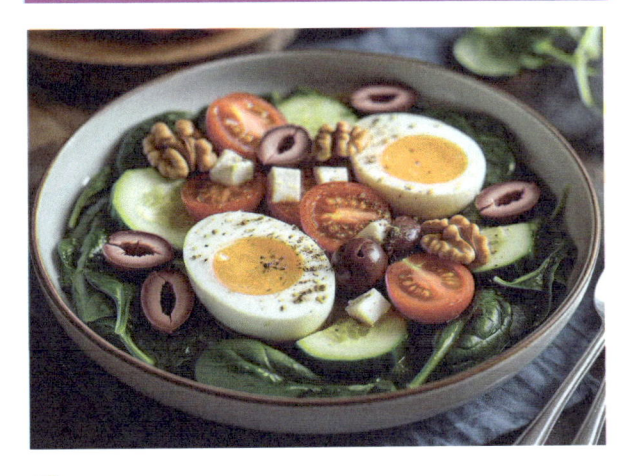

servings: 2

Ingredients

- 4 large eggs
- 1 cup (150 g) cherry tomatoes, halved
- 1/2 cup (70 g) pitted Kalamata olives, halved
- 1/2 cup (60 g) cucumber, diced
- 1/4 cup (30 g) raw walnuts, roughly chopped
- 2 cups (60 g) baby spinach, packed
- 2 tablespoons (30 ml) extra-virgin olive oil
- 1 tablespoon (15 ml) fresh lemon juice
- 1/2 teaspoon (1.5 g) fine sea salt, divided
- 1/4 teaspoon (0.5 g) ground black pepper
- 1/2 teaspoon (1 g) dried oregano
- Optional: 1/4 cup (35 g) crumbled sheep's milk feta (omit for dairy-free)
- Optional swaps: Use green olives instead of Kalamata; swap walnuts for pumpkin seeds for nut-free; use arugula instead of spinach for a peppery flavor

Directions

1. Bring a medium saucepan of water to a gentle boil over medium-high heat
2. Carefully lower eggs into boiling water using a spoon
3. Boil eggs for 7–8 minutes for medium-set yolks
4. While eggs cook, combine cherry tomatoes, olives, cucumber, and walnuts in a medium bowl
5. Add 1 tablespoon olive oil, lemon juice, 1/4 teaspoon salt, black pepper, and oregano; toss to combine
6. In a large skillet, heat remaining 1 tablespoon olive oil over medium heat
7. Add baby spinach and sauté for 1–2 minutes until just wilted; season with remaining 1/4 teaspoon salt
8. When eggs are done, transfer to a bowl of ice water for 2 minutes to stop cooking
9. Peel eggs and slice each in half
10. To assemble, divide sautéed spinach between two bowls
11. Top each with tomato-olive-walnut mixture and two halved eggs
12. Sprinkle with feta if using
13. Serve immediately

Estimated total time

Prep time: 10 minutes
Cook time: 8 minutes
Total: 18 minutes

Nutritional facts per serving

Calories: 340
Protein: 15 g
Fat: 27 g
Carbs: 13 g
Fiber: 4 g
Sugar: 4 g

Dietary labels/tags

Gluten-free
Dairy-free option
Vegetarian
Anti-inflammatory
Low-carb
Gentle-digestion
Meal-prep friendly

Suggested cooking method/program

Stovetop, boiling, sautéing

Storage & meal prep tips

Store all components separately in airtight containers in the fridge up to 3 days
Assemble just before serving for best texture
Eggs can be boiled ahead and kept unpeeled in the fridge up to 4 days
Not recommended for freezing

Cortisol reset tip

Walnuts and extra-virgin olive oil provide omega-3s and polyphenols to help lower inflammation and support healthy cortisol balance, while Mediterranean flavors promote satisfaction and mindful eating.

Possible variations

Add a handful of microgreens or fresh parsley for extra phytonutrients
Swap walnuts for sliced almonds or pumpkin seeds
Top with a spoonful of hummus for extra creaminess
Use roasted red peppers instead of tomatoes for a different flavor profile

GRAIN-FREE AND LOW-GRAIN RECIPES

30. Cauliflower Hash with Turmeric Eggs

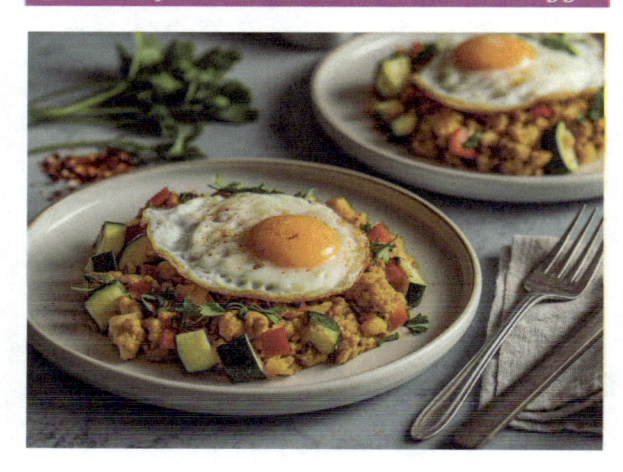

servings: 2

Ingredients

- 3 cups (300 g) cauliflower florets, riced (about 1 small head)
- 1 small red bell pepper, diced (about 3/4 cup/90 g)
- 1 small zucchini, diced (about 1 cup/120 g)
- 2 tablespoons (30 ml) extra-virgin olive oil, divided
- 1/2 teaspoon (2 g) ground turmeric, divided
- 1/2 teaspoon (2 g) smoked paprika
- 1/2 teaspoon (1.5 g) fine sea salt, divided
- 1/4 teaspoon (0.5 g) ground black pepper
- 4 large eggs
- 2 tablespoons (8 g) fresh parsley or cilantro, chopped
- Optional: 1/4 teaspoon (1 g) crushed red pepper flakes
- Optional swaps: Use broccoli rice instead of cauliflower for variety; swap zucchini for yellow squash; for low-FODMAP, use only green tops of scallions instead of bell pepper

Directions

1. Add cauliflower florets to a food processor and pulse until rice-sized pieces form; set aside
2. Heat 1 tablespoon olive oil in a large nonstick skillet over medium heat
3. Add diced bell pepper and zucchini; sauté for 3–4 minutes until just softened
4. Stir in riced cauliflower, 1/4 teaspoon salt, smoked paprika, and black pepper; cook for 5–6 minutes, stirring occasionally, until cauliflower is tender and starting to brown
5. Push hash to one side of the skillet; add remaining 1 tablespoon olive oil to the empty side
6. Crack eggs directly into the skillet, sprinkle with 1/4 teaspoon turmeric and remaining 1/4 teaspoon salt
7. Cook eggs to desired doneness, 3–4 minutes for sunny-side up or flip for over-easy
8. Sprinkle hash and eggs with fresh parsley or cilantro and red pepper flakes if using
9. Divide hash and eggs between two plates and serve hot

Estimated total time

Prep time: 10 minutes
Cook time: 15 minutes
Total: 25 minutes

Nutritional facts per serving

Calories: 260
Protein: 13 g
Fat: 18 g
Carbs: 13 g
Fiber: 4 g
Sugar: 5 g

Dietary labels/tags

Grain-free
Gluten-free

Dairy-free
Vegetarian
Anti-inflammatory
Low-carb
Gentle-digestion
Meal-prep friendly

Suggested cooking method/program

Stovetop, one-pan

Storage & meal prep tips

Store cooled hash and eggs separately in airtight containers in the fridge up to 3 days
Reheat hash in a skillet over medium heat; eggs are best cooked fresh, but can be reheated gently if needed
Not recommended for freezing

Cortisol reset tip

Turmeric and cruciferous cauliflower provide anti-inflammatory phytonutrients to help regulate cortisol and support detoxification, while eggs offer steady protein for hormone balance.

Possible variations

Top with sliced avocado for extra healthy fats
Add a handful of baby spinach to the hash for more greens
Swap eggs for tofu scramble for a vegan option. Sprinkle with hemp seeds or pumpkin seeds for added crunch and omega-3s

31. Almond Flour Blueberry Pancakes with Cinnamon

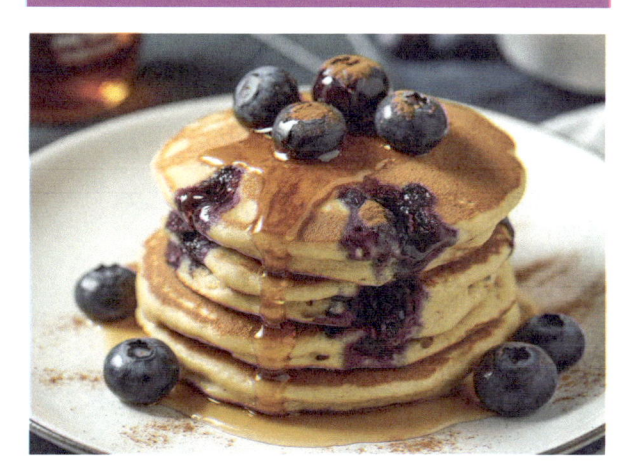

servings: 2

Ingredients

- 1 cup (96 g) blanched almond flour
- 2 large eggs
- 1/4 cup (60 ml) unsweetened almond milk
- 1 tablespoon (15 ml) pure maple syrup
- 1 teaspoon (5 ml) vanilla extract
- 1/2 teaspoon (2 g) baking powder (aluminum-free)
- 1/2 teaspoon (1.5 g) ground cinnamon
- 1/8 teaspoon (0.5 g) fine sea salt
- 1/2 cup (75 g) fresh blueberries
- 1 tablespoon (14 g) coconut oil or avocado oil, for cooking
- Optional swaps: Use coconut milk instead of almond milk for nut-free; swap blueberries for raspberries or diced strawberries; omit maple syrup for lower sugar

Directions

1. In a medium bowl, whisk together almond flour, baking powder, cinnamon, and salt
2. In a separate bowl, whisk eggs, almond milk, maple syrup, and vanilla extract until smooth
3. Pour wet ingredients into dry ingredients and stir until just combined; do not overmix
4. Gently fold in blueberries
5. Heat a large nonstick skillet or griddle over medium-low heat and add half the coconut oil
6. Once hot, scoop batter by 1/4 cup (60 ml) portions onto skillet, spacing apart
7. Cook 2–3 minutes until edges look set and bottoms are golden; flip carefully and cook another 2–3 minutes
8. Repeat with remaining batter, adding more oil as needed
9. Serve warm, optionally with extra blueberries or a drizzle of maple syrup

Estimated total time

Prep time: 8 minutes
Cook time: 12 minutes
Total: 20 minutes

Nutritional facts per serving

Calories: 320
Protein: 11 g
Fat: 24 g
Carbs: 18 g
Fiber: 4 g
Sugar: 7 g

Dietary labels/tags

Grain-free
Gluten-free
Dairy-free
Vegetarian
Anti-inflammatory
Low-carb option
Gentle-digestion

Suggested cooking method/program

Stovetop, skillet or griddle

Storage & meal prep tips

Store cooled pancakes in an airtight container in the fridge up to 3 days
Reheat gently in a toaster oven or skillet over low heat
Freeze in a single layer, then transfer to a freezer bag for up to 2 months; reheat from frozen in toaster

Cortisol reset tip

Almond flour and blueberries provide antioxidants and healthy fats to help reduce inflammation and support steady energy, while cinnamon helps balance blood sugar and cortisol response.

Possible variations

Add 1 tablespoon ground flaxseed for extra fiber
Top with a dollop of coconut yogurt for probiotics
Swap blueberries for chopped apples and add a pinch of nutmeg
Make mini pancakes for a fun, kid-friendly option

32. Savory Zucchini & Egg Muffin Cups with Sunflower Seeds

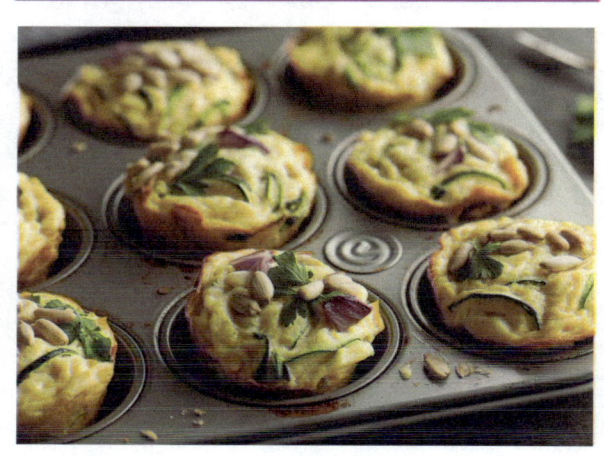

servings: 4

Ingredients

- 1 1/2 cups (180 g) grated zucchini (about 1 medium)
- 4 large eggs
- 1/4 cup (60 ml) unsweetened almond milk
- 1/3 cup (40 g) finely diced red onion
- 1/4 cup (30 g) chopped fresh parsley
- 1/4 cup (32 g) raw sunflower seeds
- 1/2 teaspoon (2 g) fine sea salt
- 1/4 teaspoon (0.5 g) ground black pepper
- 1/2 teaspoon (1 g) garlic powder
- 1/2 teaspoon (1 g) dried oregano
- 1 tablespoon (15 ml) extra-virgin olive oil, for greasing
- Optional swaps: Use coconut milk for nut-free; swap red onion for green onion for low-FODMAP; use pumpkin seeds instead of sunflower seeds

Directions

1. Preheat oven to 350°F (175°C). Grease a 12-cup muffin tin with olive oil or line with silicone liners
2. Place grated zucchini in a clean kitchen towel and squeeze out as much moisture as possible
3. In a large bowl, whisk eggs, almond milk, salt, pepper, garlic powder, and oregano until well combined
4. Stir in zucchini, red onion, parsley, and sunflower seeds
5. Divide mixture evenly among 8 muffin cups (about 1/4 cup per cup)
6. Bake for 22–25 minutes, until muffins are set and lightly golden on top
7. Let cool in pan for 5 minutes, then run a knife around edges and remove
8. Serve warm or at room temperature

Estimated total time

Prep time: 10 minutes
Cook time: 25 minutes
Total: 35 minutes

Nutritional facts per serving

Calories: 120
Protein: 7 g
Fat: 8 g
Carbs: 5 g
Fiber: 1 g
Sugar: 2 g

Dietary labels/tags

Grain-free
Gluten-free
Dairy-free
Vegetarian
Anti-inflammatory
Low-carb
Meal-prep friendly
Gentle-digestion

Suggested cooking method/program

Oven, muffin tin

Storage & meal prep tips

Store cooled muffin cups in an airtight container in the fridge up to 4 days
Reheat in microwave for 20–30 seconds or in a toaster oven at 300°F for 5 minutes
Freeze in a single layer, then transfer to a freezer bag for up to 2 months; thaw overnight in fridge before reheating

Cortisol reset tip

Sunflower seeds and zucchini provide magnesium and antioxidants to help regulate stress response and support hormone balance, while eggs offer steady protein for sustained energy.

Possible variations

Add 1/4 cup (30 g) chopped spinach or kale for extra greens
Sprinkle with hemp seeds or pumpkin seeds for a nut-free crunch
Mix in 1/4 cup (30 g) crumbled feta for a tangy flavor (if dairy is tolerated)

33. Warm Hemp-Seed Porridge with Cinnamon & Pear

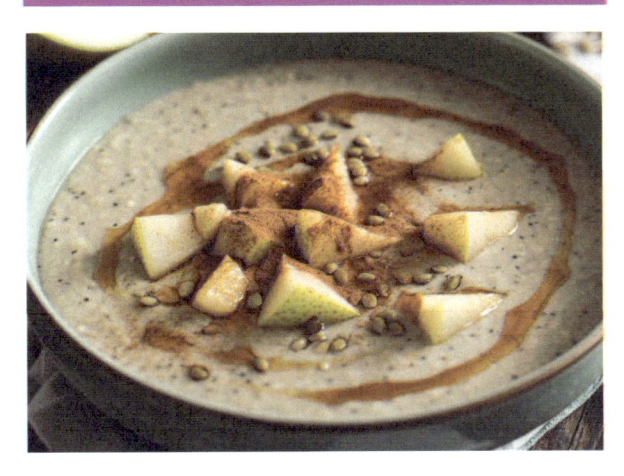

servings: 2

Ingredients

- 1/2 cup (80 g) hulled hemp seeds (hemp hearts)
- 1 cup (240 ml) unsweetened almond milk
- 1/2 cup (120 ml) water
- 1 medium ripe pear, diced (about 140 g)
- 1 tablespoon (15 ml) pure maple syrup
- 1 teaspoon (2 g) ground cinnamon
- 1/4 teaspoon (1 g) ground ginger
- 1/8 teaspoon (0.5 g) fine sea salt
- 1 teaspoon (5 ml) vanilla extract
- 1 tablespoon (10 g) chia seeds
- Optional swaps: Use coconut milk for nut-free; swap pear for apple or berries; omit maple syrup for lower sugar; use ground flaxseed instead of chia seeds

Directions

1. In a small saucepan, combine hemp seeds, almond milk, water, cinnamon, ginger, and salt
2. Bring to a gentle simmer over medium heat, stirring frequently
3. Add diced pear and continue to cook for 5–6 minutes, stirring occasionally, until pear is softened and mixture thickens
4. Stir in chia seeds, vanilla extract, and maple syrup
5. Cook for 1–2 more minutes, stirring, until porridge reaches desired consistency
6. Remove from heat and let sit 1 minute to thicken further
7. Divide between two bowls and serve warm, optionally topped with extra pear, a sprinkle of cinnamon, or a few hemp seeds

Estimated total time

Prep time: 5 minutes
Cook time: 7 minutes
Total: 12 minutes

Nutritional facts per serving

Calories: 310
Protein: 11 g
Fat: 20 g
Carbs: 22 g
Fiber: 6 g
Sugar: 10 g

Dietary labels/tags

Grain-free
Gluten-free
Dairy-free
Vegan-friendly
Anti-inflammatory
Low-glycemic
Gentle-digestion

Suggested cooking method/program

Stovetop, saucepan

Storage & meal prep tips

Store cooled porridge in an airtight container in the fridge up to 3 days

Reheat gently in a saucepan over low heat, adding a splash of almond milk to loosen if needed
Not recommended for freezing due to texture changes

Cortisol reset tip

Hemp seeds and chia seeds provide plant-based omega-3s and magnesium to help lower inflammation and support balanced cortisol, while cinnamon helps stabilize blood sugar for steady energy.

Possible variations

Add 1 tablespoon almond butter for extra creaminess
Top with chopped walnuts or pecans for crunch
Stir in 1/4 cup (30 g) blueberries or raspberries for a berry twist
Use unsweetened applesauce instead of pear for a smoother texture

34. Sweet Potato Avocado Skillet with Poached Eggs

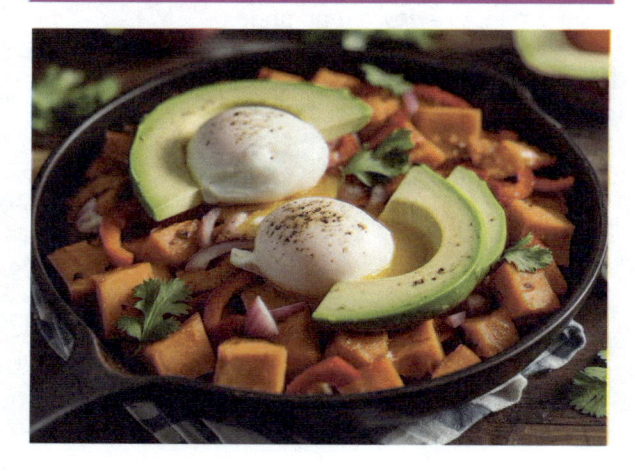

servings: 2

Ingredients

- 1 medium sweet potato (about 8 oz/225 g), peeled and diced into 1/2-inch cubes
- 1 tablespoon (15 ml) extra-virgin olive oil
- 1/2 teaspoon (2 g) fine sea salt
- 1/4 teaspoon (0.5 g) ground black pepper
- 1/2 teaspoon (1 g) smoked paprika
- 1/2 teaspoon (1 g) ground cumin
- 1 small red bell pepper (about 4 oz/115 g), diced
- 1/4 cup (40 g) finely diced red onion
- 1 ripe avocado (about 6 oz/170 g), peeled, pitted, and sliced
- 4 large eggs
- 2 tablespoons (8 g) chopped fresh cilantro or parsley
- 1 tablespoon (15 ml) apple cider vinegar (for poaching eggs)
- Optional swaps: Use white potato for low-FODMAP; swap red onion for green onion; omit avocado for lower fat; use ghee instead of olive oil

Directions

1. Bring a medium saucepan of water to a gentle simmer (not boiling) and add apple cider vinegar
2. Heat olive oil in a large nonstick or cast-iron skillet over medium heat
3. Add diced sweet potato, salt, pepper, smoked paprika, and cumin
4. Sauté for 6–7 minutes, stirring occasionally, until sweet potato begins to soften
5. Add red bell pepper and red onion to the skillet
6. Continue to cook for 5–6 minutes, stirring, until vegetables are tender and sweet potato is golden
7. While vegetables cook, crack each egg into a small bowl
8. Swirl simmering water with a spoon to create a gentle whirlpool, then carefully slide in eggs one at a time
9. Poach eggs for 3–4 minutes, until whites are set but yolks are still runny
10. Use a slotted spoon to remove eggs and drain on a paper towel
11. Divide sweet potato mixture between two plates
12. Top each with sliced avocado and two poached eggs
13. Sprinkle with chopped cilantro or parsley and extra black pepper if desired

Estimated total time

Prep time: 10 minutes
Cook time: 18 minutes
Total: 28 minutes

Nutritional facts per serving

Calories: 340
Protein: 13 g
Fat: 20 g
Carbs: 29 g
Fiber: 7 g
Sugar: 6 g

Dietary labels/tags

Grain-free
Gluten-free

Dairy-free
Vegetarian
Anti-inflammatory
Low-glycemic
Gentle-digestion

Suggested cooking method/program

Stovetop, skillet and saucepan

Storage & meal prep tips

Store cooked sweet potato mixture in an airtight container in the fridge up to 3 days
Poach eggs fresh for best texture; reheat sweet potato mixture in a skillet over medium heat for 3–4 minutes
Avocado should be sliced fresh before serving; do not freeze

Cortisol reset tip

Sweet potatoes provide slow-digesting carbs and vitamin C to help regulate cortisol, while avocado and eggs offer healthy fats and protein for steady energy and hormone support.

Possible variations

Add 1/2 cup (75 g) baby spinach or kale to the skillet for extra greens
Top with a sprinkle of hemp seeds or pumpkin seeds for crunch
Use roasted butternut squash instead of sweet potato for a fall twist
Add a dash of hot sauce or red pepper flakes for gentle heat

FAMILY-FRIENDLY GRAB-AND-GO: 5 RECIPES

35. Berry-Kefir Overnight Oats with Flax

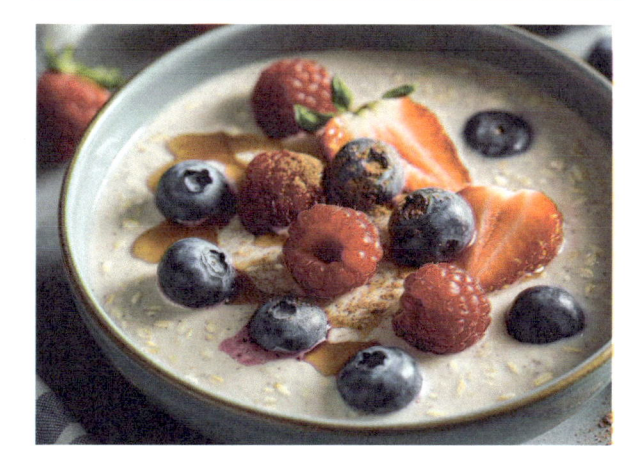

servings: 2

Ingredients

- 1 cup (80 g) old-fashioned rolled oats (certified gluten-free if needed)
- 1 cup (240 ml) plain unsweetened kefir (dairy or coconut-based for dairy-free)
- 1/2 cup (120 ml) unsweetened almond milk
- 1 tablespoon (10 g) ground flaxseed
- 1 cup (140 g) mixed fresh or frozen berries (blueberries, raspberries, strawberries)
- 1 tablespoon (15 ml) pure maple syrup
- 1/2 teaspoon (2 g) ground cinnamon
- 1/2 teaspoon (2 ml) vanilla extract
- Pinch fine sea salt
- Optional swaps: Use oat milk for nut-free; swap flaxseed for chia seeds; omit maple syrup for lower sugar; use all blueberries for low-FODMAP

Directions

1. In a medium glass jar or container, combine oats, kefir, almond milk, ground flaxseed, cinnamon, vanilla extract, and salt
2. Stir well to fully incorporate all ingredients
3. Fold in mixed berries and drizzle with maple syrup
4. Cover tightly and refrigerate for at least 6 hours or overnight
5. In the morning, stir oats well and divide between two bowls or jars
6. Top with extra berries or a sprinkle of flaxseed if desired

Estimated total time

Prep time: 8 minutes
Chill time: 6–8 hours (overnight)
Total: 8 hours 8 minutes

Nutritional facts per serving

Calories: 260
Protein: 9 g
Fat: 6 g
Carbs: 42 g
Fiber: 7 g
Sugar: 11 g

Dietary labels/tags

Gluten-free (if using certified oats)
Dairy-free option
Vegetarian
Anti-inflammatory

Low-glycemic
Gentle-digestion

Suggested cooking method/program

No-cook, overnight refrigeration

Storage & meal prep tips

Store in an airtight container in the fridge up to 3 days
Stir before serving; add a splash of almond milk if too thick
Not recommended for freezing due to texture changes

Cortisol reset tip

Kefir provides probiotics to support gut health and lower inflammation, while flaxseed and berries deliver fiber and antioxidants for balanced blood sugar and steady energy.

Possible variations

Add 2 tablespoons chopped walnuts or pecans for crunch
Stir in 1/4 cup (60 g) unsweetened applesauce for extra creaminess
Top with pumpkin seeds or hemp hearts for added protein

36. Savory Spinach & Feta Egg Muffins with Pumpkin Seeds

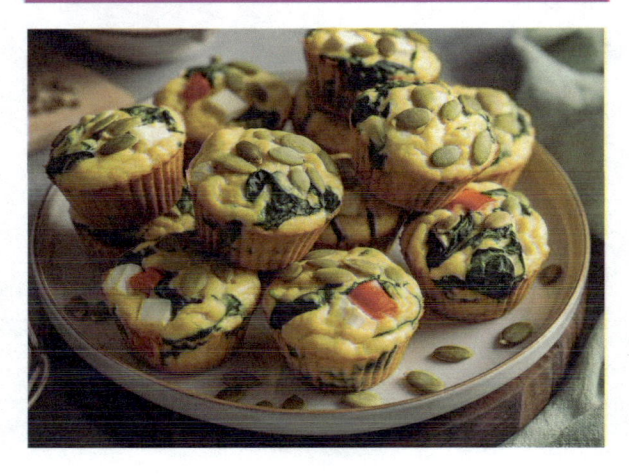

servings: 6 (makes 12 muffins)

Ingredients

- 8 large eggs
- 1/3 cup (80 ml) unsweetened almond milk
- 1/2 teaspoon (2 g) fine sea salt
- 1/4 teaspoon (0.5 g) ground black pepper
- 1/2 teaspoon (1 g) dried oregano
- 2 cups (60 g) baby spinach, finely chopped
- 1/2 cup (75 g) crumbled feta cheese (use dairy-free feta for dairy-free)
- 1/4 cup (30 g) diced red bell pepper
- 1/4 cup (30 g) thinly sliced green onion
- 1/4 cup (30 g) raw pumpkin seeds (pepitas)
- 1 tablespoon (15 ml) extra-virgin olive oil (for greasing muffin tin)
- Optional swaps: Use coconut milk for nut-free; swap feta for goat cheese or omit for dairy-free; use kale instead of spinach; omit onion for low-FODMAP

Directions

1. Preheat oven to 350°F (175°C).
2. Lightly grease a standard 12-cup muffin tin with olive oil or line with silicone muffin liners.
3. In a large mixing bowl, whisk eggs, almond milk, salt, pepper, and oregano until well combined.
4. Stir in chopped spinach, feta, red bell pepper, and green onion.
5. Evenly divide the egg mixture among the 12 muffin cups, filling each about 3/4 full.
6. Sprinkle pumpkin seeds evenly over the tops of each muffin.
7. Bake for 20–22 minutes, until muffins are puffed and set in the center.
8. Let cool in the pan for 5 minutes, then run a thin spatula around edges and remove muffins.
9. Serve warm or at room temperature.

Estimated total time

Prep time: 10 minutes
Cook time: 22 minutes
Total: 32 minutes

Nutritional facts per serving

Calories: 120
Protein: 8 g
Fat: 8 g
Carbs: 3 g
Fiber: 1 g
Sugar: 1 g

Dietary labels/tags

Gluten-free

Vegetarian
Dairy-free option
Low-glycemic
Anti-inflammatory
Meal-prep friendly

Suggested cooking method/program

Oven-baked, muffin tin

Storage & meal prep tips

Store cooled muffins in an airtight container in the fridge up to 4 days
Reheat in the microwave for 30–40 seconds or enjoy cold
Freeze up to 2 months; thaw overnight in the fridge before reheating

Cortisol reset tip

Eggs and pumpkin seeds provide protein and magnesium to help stabilize blood sugar and support healthy cortisol rhythms, while spinach delivers anti-inflammatory phytonutrients.

Possible variations

Add 1/2 cup (75 g) chopped mushrooms or zucchini for extra veggies
Top with a sprinkle of hemp hearts for more omega-3s
Use sun-dried tomatoes instead of bell pepper for a Mediterranean twist
Swap feta for shredded cheddar or omit cheese for dairy-free

37. Almond-Butter Banana Chia Wrap

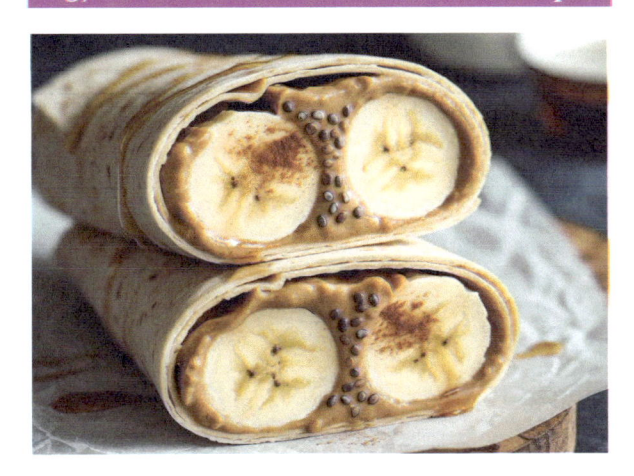

servings: 2

Ingredients

- 2 large gluten-free tortillas (about 8-inch/20 cm each)
- 4 tablespoons (64 g) unsweetened almond butter
- 1 medium ripe banana, sliced (about 120 g)
- 2 teaspoons (10 g) chia seeds
- 1 tablespoon (15 ml) pure maple syrup
- 1/4 teaspoon (1 g) ground cinnamon
- Pinch fine sea salt
- Optional swaps: Use sunflower seed butter for nut-free; swap maple syrup for raw honey or omit for lower sugar; use coconut wraps for grain-free; use low-FODMAP tortilla if needed

Directions

1. Lay tortillas flat on a clean surface or cutting board
2. Spread 2 tablespoons almond butter evenly over each tortilla, leaving a 1/2-inch border
3. Arrange banana slices in a single layer down the center of each tortilla
4. Sprinkle 1 teaspoon chia seeds, 1/8 teaspoon cinnamon, and a pinch of salt over the banana on each wrap
5. Drizzle 1/2 tablespoon maple syrup over the filling in each wrap
6. Tightly roll up each tortilla from one side, tucking in the ends as you go to form a secure wrap
7. Slice each wrap in half on the diagonal and serve immediately, or wrap tightly in parchment for grab-and-go

Estimated total time

Prep time: 7 minutes
No cook time
Total: 7 minutes

Nutritional facts per serving

Calories: 270
Protein: 7 g
Fat: 13 g
Carbs: 34 g
Fiber: 6 g
Sugar: 10 g

Dietary labels/tags

Gluten-free (with GF tortillas)
Dairy-free
Vegan
Anti-inflammatory
Low-glycemic option
Nut-free option

Suggested cooking method/program

No-cook, assembly only

Storage & meal prep tips

Wrap tightly in parchment or foil and refrigerate up to 24 hours
Best enjoyed fresh; banana may brown slightly if stored longer
Not recommended for freezing

Cortisol reset tip

Almond butter and chia seeds provide healthy fats and magnesium to help stabilize blood sugar and support calm energy, while bananas offer potassium for gentle adrenal support.

Possible variations

Add 2 tablespoons unsweetened coconut flakes for extra texture
Swap banana for sliced strawberries or blueberries
Spread a thin layer of coconut yogurt before adding fruit for extra creaminess. Sprinkle with hemp hearts or pumpkin seeds for added protein and crunch

38. Sweet Potato & Apple Breakfast Hand Pies with Walnuts

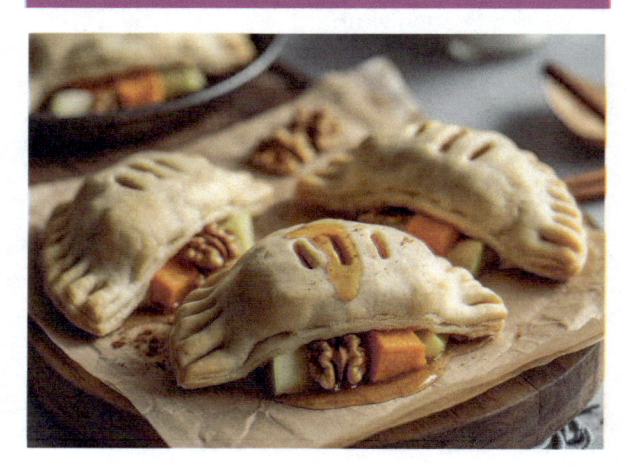

servings: 4 (makes 4 hand pies)

Ingredients

- 1 medium sweet potato (about 8 oz/225 g), peeled and diced
- 1 medium apple (about 6 oz/170 g), peeled, cored, and diced
- 1 tablespoon (15 ml) coconut oil, melted
- ½ teaspoon (1 g) ground cinnamon
- ¼ teaspoon (0.5 g) ground ginger
- 1/8 teaspoon (0.25 g) fine sea salt
- 2 tablespoons (30 ml) pure maple syrup
- 1/3 cup (35 g) chopped raw walnuts
- 1 teaspoon (5 ml) fresh lemon juice
- 1 package (7 oz/200 g) gluten-free pie crust dough (store-bought or homemade)
- 1 egg, beaten (for egg wash; omit for vegan and use plant milk)
- Optional swaps: Use pecans instead of walnuts; swap coconut oil for avocado oil; use a dairy-free/vegan pie crust; use pear instead of apple; omit nuts for nut-free

Directions

1. Preheat oven to 375°F (190°C). Line a baking sheet with parchment paper.
2. Place diced sweet potato in a small saucepan, cover with water, and bring to a boil. Simmer for 8–10 minutes until fork-tender. Drain well and transfer to a mixing bowl.
3. Add diced apple, melted coconut oil, cinnamon, ginger, sea salt, maple syrup, walnuts, and lemon juice to the bowl. Stir to combine.
4. On a lightly floured surface, roll out the pie crust dough to about 1/8-inch thickness. Cut into 8 circles, each about 4 inches (10 cm) in diameter.
5. Spoon about 2 heaping tablespoons of filling onto the center of 4 circles, leaving a ½-inch border.
6. Top each with a second dough circle. Press edges together with a fork to seal.
7. Brush tops with beaten egg or plant milk. Cut a small slit in the top of each hand pie for steam to escape.
8. Place hand pies on the prepared baking sheet.
9. Bake for 20–25 minutes, until golden brown and crisp.
10. Cool on the baking sheet for 5 minutes before serving warm or at room temperature.

Estimated total time

Prep time: 15 minutes
Cook time: 25 minutes
Total: 40 minutes

Nutritional facts per serving

Calories: 260
Protein: 4 g
Fat: 13 g
Carbs: 34 g
Fiber: 3 g
Sugar: 10 g

Dietary labels/tags

Gluten-free (with GF crust)
Vegetarian
Dairy-free option

Vegan option
Anti-inflammatory
Nut-free option

Suggested cooking method/program

Oven-baked, hand pies

Storage & meal prep tips

Store cooled hand pies in an airtight container at room temperature for up to 24 hours or refrigerate up to 3 days
Reheat in a toaster oven at 325°F (165°C) for 5–7 minutes
Freeze unbaked hand pies for up to 1 month; bake from frozen, adding 5 minutes to cook time

Cortisol reset tip

Sweet potatoes and walnuts provide complex carbs and magnesium to help stabilize blood sugar and support healthy cortisol balance, while cinnamon and ginger offer anti-inflammatory benefits.

Possible variations

Add 2 tablespoons (20 g) dried cranberries for a tart twist
Swap apple for pear or diced ripe peach
Sprinkle with hemp hearts before baking for extra omega-3s
Use sunflower seeds instead of walnuts for a nut-free version

39. Citrus-Ginger Hemp Yogurt Jars

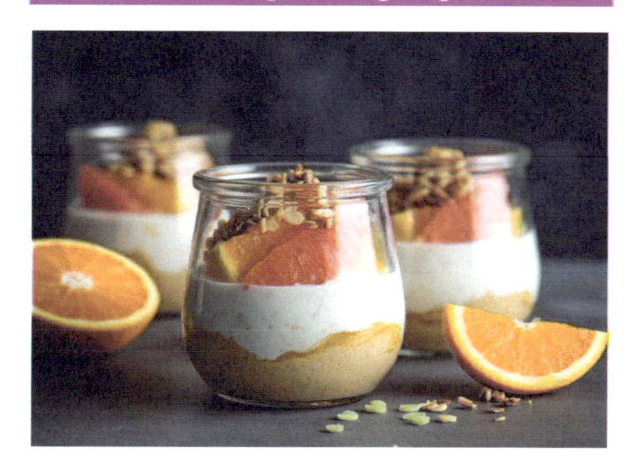

servings: 2

Ingredients

- 1 cup (240 g) unsweetened coconut yogurt
- 1 medium orange, peeled and segmented (about 130 g)
- 1/2 medium grapefruit, peeled and segmented (about 90 g)
- 2 tablespoons (20 g) shelled hemp hearts
- 1 tablespoon (15 ml) pure maple syrup
- 1/2 teaspoon (2 g) freshly grated ginger
- 1/2 teaspoon (2 g) orange zest
- 1/4 teaspoon (1 g) ground turmeric
- 1/4 cup (30 g) gluten-free granola (optional, for topping)
- Pinch fine sea salt
- Optional swaps: Use almond or cashew yogurt for nut-based; swap maple syrup for raw honey; use only orange or only grapefruit; omit granola for grain-free; use low-FODMAP yogurt if needed

Directions

1. In a medium bowl, whisk together coconut yogurt, grated ginger, orange zest, turmeric, maple syrup, and a pinch of sea salt until smooth
2. Divide half the yogurt mixture evenly between two 8-ounce (240 ml) jars or containers
3. Layer half the orange and grapefruit segments over the yogurt in each jar
4. Sprinkle 1 tablespoon hemp hearts over the fruit in each jar
5. Repeat with remaining yogurt, then top with remaining citrus segments
6. If using, sprinkle 2 tablespoons granola on top of each jar just before serving
7. Seal jars and refrigerate until ready to eat, up to 2 days

Estimated total time

Prep time: 10 minutes
No cook time
Total: 10 minutes

Nutritional facts per serving

Calories: 210
Protein: 6 g
Fat: 10 g
Carbs: 27 g
Fiber: 4 g
Sugar: 14 g

Dietary labels/tags

Gluten-free
Dairy-free
Vegan
Anti-inflammatory
Grain-free option
Low-glycemic option

Suggested cooking method/program

No-cook, assembly only

Storage & meal prep tips

Seal jars tightly and refrigerate up to 2 days
Add granola just before serving to keep it crisp
Not recommended for freezing

Cortisol reset tip

Hemp hearts and coconut yogurt provide plant-based protein and healthy fats to help stabilize blood sugar and support adrenal health, while ginger and citrus offer anti-inflammatory and immune-boosting benefits.

Possible variations

Swap grapefruit for diced kiwi or pineapple for a sweeter twist
Add 2 tablespoons unsweetened shredded coconut for extra texture
Stir in 1 tablespoon chia seeds for added fiber and omega-3s
Use plain Greek yogurt (if not dairy-free) for extra protein

SATISFYING LUNCHES

FRESH SALADS AND NOURISH BOWLS

40. Kale Quinoa Citrus Detox Salad

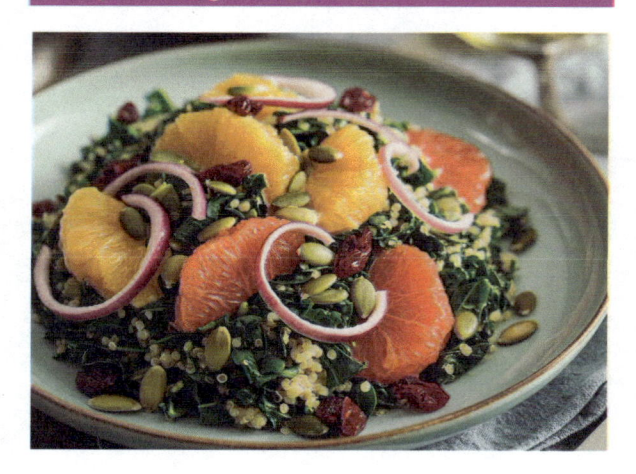

servings: 4

Ingredients

- 1 cup (170 g) uncooked quinoa, rinsed
- 2 cups (480 ml) water
- 1 medium bunch lacinato kale (about 6 oz/170 g), stems removed, leaves finely chopped
- 1 large orange, peeled and segmented, cut into bite-size pieces (about 6 oz/170 g)
- 1 medium pink grapefruit, peeled and segmented, cut into bite-size pieces (about 7 oz/200 g)
- 1/2 small red onion (about 2 oz/55 g), thinly sliced
- 1/3 cup (40 g) raw pumpkin seeds (pepitas)
- 1/4 cup (35 g) dried unsweetened cranberries
- 1/4 cup (60 ml) extra-virgin olive oil
- 2 tablespoons (30 ml) fresh lemon juice
- 1 tablespoon (15 ml) pure maple syrup
- 1 teaspoon (5 ml) Dijon mustard
- 1/2 teaspoon (2 g) fine sea salt
- 1/4 teaspoon (0.5 g) ground black pepper
- Optional swaps: Use baby kale or baby spinach instead of lacinato kale; swap pumpkin seeds for sunflower seeds; use lime juice instead of lemon; omit onion for low-FODMAP; use golden raisins instead of cranberries

Directions

1. In a medium saucepan, combine quinoa and water. Bring to a boil over high heat, then reduce heat to low, cover, and simmer for 12–15 minutes until water is absorbed and quinoa is tender. Remove from heat, fluff with a fork, and let cool for 5 minutes.
2. While quinoa cooks, place chopped kale in a large salad bowl. Sprinkle with a pinch of salt and massage with clean hands for 1–2 minutes until leaves soften and darken.
3. In a small bowl or jar, whisk together olive oil, lemon juice, maple syrup, Dijon mustard, sea salt, and black pepper until emulsified.
4. Add cooled quinoa, orange segments, grapefruit segments, red onion, pumpkin seeds, and cranberries to the kale.
5. Drizzle dressing over the salad and toss well to combine.
6. Taste and adjust seasoning if needed. Serve immediately or refrigerate up to 2 hours before serving for flavors to meld.

Estimated total time

Prep time: 15 minutes
Cook time: 15 minutes
Total: 30 minutes

Nutritional facts per serving

Calories: 320
Protein: 8 g
Fat: 15 g
Carbs: 41 g
Fiber: 6 g
Sugar: 11 g

Dietary labels/tags

Gluten-free
Dairy-free
Vegan
Anti-inflammatory
Nut-free
Low-glycemic option

Suggested cooking method/program

Stovetop (quinoa), no-cook assembly

Storage & meal prep tips

Store salad in an airtight container in the refrigerator for up to 3 days
If making ahead, keep dressing separate and toss just before serving for best texture
Not recommended for freezing

Cortisol reset tip

Kale and citrus fruits are rich in vitamin C and antioxidants that help lower inflammation and support adrenal health, while quinoa provides steady energy to help balance cortisol.

Possible variations

Add 1/2 avocado, diced, for extra creaminess
Top with 1/4 cup (30 g) crumbled feta (if not dairy-free)
Swap grapefruit for 1 cup (150 g) diced strawberries in spring
Add 1/2 cup (80 g) cooked chickpeas for extra plant protein

41. Turmeric-Grilled Chicken & Roasted Sweet Potato Nourish Bowl

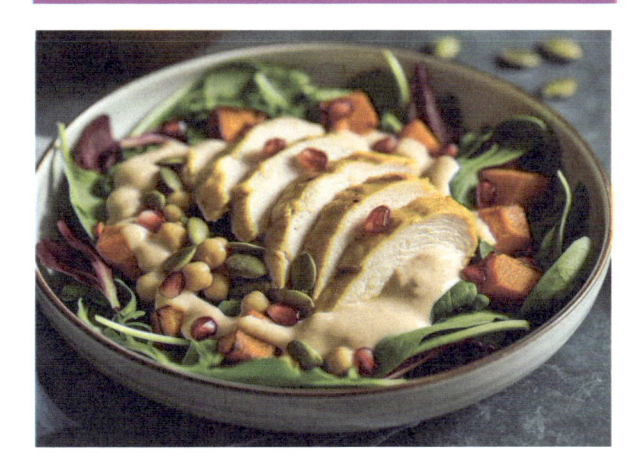

servings: 2

Ingredients

- 2 medium boneless, skinless chicken breasts (about 12 oz/340 g total)
- 2 tablespoons (30 ml) extra-virgin olive oil, divided
- 1 tablespoon (15 ml) fresh lemon juice
- 1 teaspoon (2 g) ground turmeric
- 1/2 teaspoon (1 g) ground cumin
- 1/2 teaspoon (1 g) smoked paprika
- 1/2 teaspoon (2 g) fine sea salt, divided
- 1/4 teaspoon (0.5 g) ground black pepper
- 2 medium sweet potatoes (about 16 oz/450 g), peeled and cut into 1/2-inch cubes
- 4 cups (120 g) mixed baby greens (spinach, arugula, or spring mix)
- 1/2 cup (80 g) cooked chickpeas, drained and rinsed
- 1/4 cup (30 g) raw pumpkin seeds (pepitas)
- 1/4 cup (35 g) pomegranate seeds (optional)
- 1/4 cup (60 ml) plain unsweetened coconut yogurt (for drizzle)
- 1 tablespoon (15 ml) water (to thin yogurt)
- 1/2 teaspoon (2 g) grated fresh ginger
- Optional swaps: Use boneless chicken thighs instead of breasts; swap sweet potatoes for butternut squash; use sunflower seeds instead of pumpkin seeds; omit pomegranate for low-FODMAP; use Greek yogurt if not dairy-free

Directions

1. Preheat oven to 425°F (220°C). Line a large baking sheet with parchment paper.
2. In a medium bowl, toss sweet potato cubes with 1 tablespoon olive oil and 1/4 teaspoon salt. Spread evenly on prepared baking sheet. Roast for 25–30 minutes, flipping halfway, until golden and tender.
3. While sweet potatoes roast, in a shallow dish, whisk together remaining 1 tablespoon olive oil, lemon juice, turmeric, cumin, smoked paprika, 1/4 teaspoon salt, and black pepper. Add chicken breasts and turn to coat. Let marinate at room temperature for 10–15 minutes.
4. Heat a grill pan or outdoor grill over medium-high heat. Grill chicken for 5–6 minutes per side, or until cooked through and internal temperature reaches 165°F (74°C). Transfer to a plate and let rest 5 minutes, then slice.
5. In a small bowl, whisk coconut yogurt, water, and grated ginger until smooth.
6. To assemble bowls, divide greens between two large bowls. Top each with half the roasted sweet potatoes, sliced chicken, chickpeas, pumpkin seeds, and pomegranate seeds (if using). Drizzle with ginger yogurt sauce.
7. Serve immediately.

Estimated total time

Prep time: 15 minutes
Cook time: 30 minutes
Total: 45 minutes

Nutritional facts per serving

Calories: 430
Protein: 32 g
Fat: 16 g
Carbs: 41 g
Fiber: 8 g
Sugar: 10 g

Dietary labels/tags

Gluten-free
Dairy-free
Anti-inflammatory
High-protein
Nut-free
Low-glycemic option

Suggested cooking method/program

Oven roasting (sweet potatoes), grill or grill pan (chicken), no-cook assembly

Storage & meal prep tips

Store components separately in airtight containers in the refrigerator for up to 3 days
Reheat sweet potatoes and chicken gently before assembling, or enjoy cold
Keep yogurt sauce in a small jar and drizzle just before serving
Not recommended for freezing

Cortisol reset tip

Turmeric and ginger are potent anti-inflammatory spices that help modulate cortisol and support immune balance, while sweet potatoes provide steady, mood-supporting complex carbs.

Possible variations

Swap chicken for grilled wild salmon or tofu for a pescatarian or vegan bowl
Add 1/2 avocado, sliced, for extra healthy fats
Use roasted cauliflower or carrots instead of sweet potatoes
Top with a sprinkle of hemp hearts for added omega-3s

42. Cucumber Mint Quinoa Tabbouleh with Pistachios

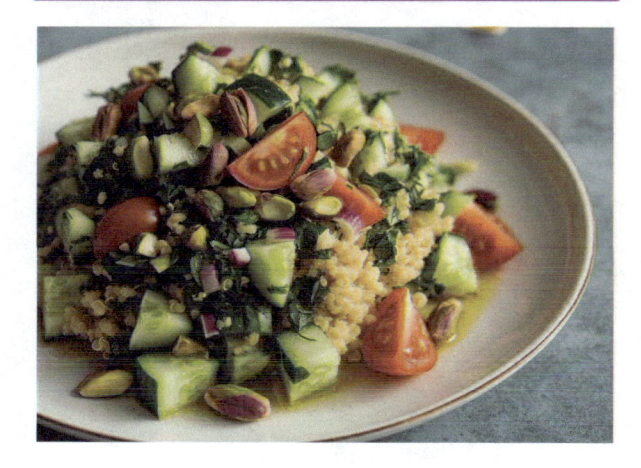

servings: 4

Ingredients

- 1 cup (170 g) uncooked quinoa, rinsed
- 2 cups (480 ml) water
- 1 1/2 cups (200 g) diced English cucumber (about 1 medium)
- 1 cup (30 g) fresh flat-leaf parsley, finely chopped
- 1/2 cup (15 g) fresh mint leaves, finely chopped
- 1/3 cup (40 g) shelled raw pistachios, roughly chopped
- 1/2 cup (80 g) cherry tomatoes, quartered
- 1/4 cup (30 g) finely diced red onion
- 1/4 cup (60 ml) extra-virgin olive oil
- 3 tablespoons (45 ml) fresh lemon juice
- 1 teaspoon (5 g) fine sea salt
- 1/4 teaspoon (0.5 g) ground black pepper
- Optional swaps: Use tri-color quinoa for extra color; swap pistachios for pumpkin seeds for nut-free; use scallions instead of red onion for milder flavor; omit tomatoes for low-FODMAP; use lime juice instead of lemon

Directions

1. In a medium saucepan, combine quinoa and water. Bring to a boil over high heat, then reduce heat to low, cover, and simmer for 12–15 minutes until water is absorbed and quinoa is tender. Remove from heat, fluff with a fork, and let cool for 5–10 minutes.
2. In a large mixing bowl, combine cooled quinoa, diced cucumber, parsley, mint, pistachios, cherry tomatoes, and red onion.
3. In a small bowl or jar, whisk together olive oil, lemon juice, sea salt, and black pepper until well combined.
4. Pour dressing over the quinoa mixture and toss thoroughly to coat all ingredients evenly.
5. Taste and adjust seasoning if needed. Serve immediately, or refrigerate for up to 2 hours to allow flavors to meld.

Estimated total time

Prep time: 15 minutes
Cook time: 15 minutes
Total: 30 minutes

Nutritional facts per serving

Calories: 310
Protein: 8 g
Fat: 16 g
Carbs: 36 g
Fiber: 5 g
Sugar: 4 g

Dietary labels/tags

Gluten-free
Dairy-free
Vegan
Anti-inflammatory
Nut-free option
Low-glycemic

Suggested cooking method/program

Stovetop (quinoa), no-cook assembly

Storage & meal prep tips

Store in an airtight container in the refrigerator for up to 3 days
Best served chilled or at room temperature
Not recommended for freezing

Cortisol reset tip

Mint and parsley are rich in antioxidants and phytonutrients that help reduce inflammation and support adrenal health, while pistachios provide healthy fats and magnesium to help regulate stress response.

Possible variations

Add 1/2 avocado, diced, for extra creaminess
Top with 1/4 cup (30 g) crumbled feta (if not dairy-free)
Swap pistachios for toasted sunflower seeds for a nut-free version
Add 1/2 cup (80 g) cooked chickpeas for extra plant protein
Use chopped dill or cilantro in place of mint for a different flavor profile

43. Miso-Glazed Tempeh & Broccoli Brown Rice Bowl

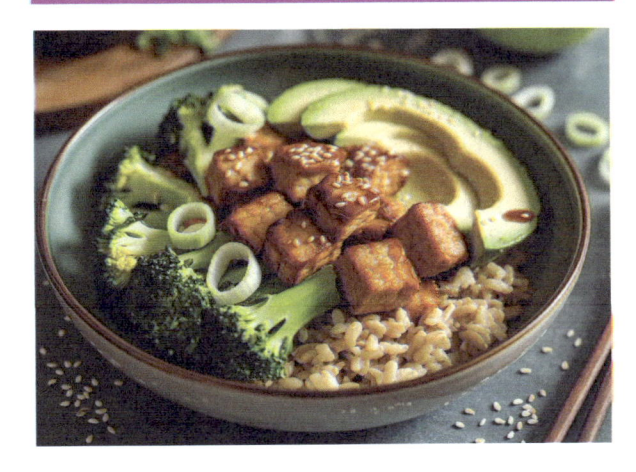

servings: 2

Ingredients

- 1/2 cup (90 g) uncooked brown rice
- 1 cup (240 ml) water
- 1 (8 oz/225 g) block organic tempeh, cut into 1/2-inch cubes
- 2 cups (140 g) broccoli florets
- 1 tablespoon (15 ml) avocado oil, divided
- 2 tablespoons (30 g) white or yellow miso paste
- 1 tablespoon (15 ml) pure maple syrup
- 1 tablespoon (15 ml) rice vinegar
- 1 tablespoon (15 ml) low-sodium tamari or coconut aminos
- 1 teaspoon (5 ml) toasted sesame oil
- 1 teaspoon (5 g) freshly grated ginger
- 1 clove garlic, minced
- 1/4 teaspoon (1 g) ground black pepper
- 1/2 small avocado, sliced
- 2 tablespoons (16 g) toasted sesame seeds
- 2 scallions, thinly sliced
- Optional swaps: Use quinoa instead of brown rice for quicker cooking; swap tempeh for extra-firm tofu; use coconut aminos for soy-free; omit garlic for low-FODMAP; use cauliflower rice for grain-free

Directions

1. Rinse brown rice under cold water. In a small saucepan, combine rice and water. Bring to a boil, reduce heat to low, cover, and simmer for 25 minutes or until water is absorbed and rice is tender. Remove from heat and let stand, covered, for 5 minutes.
2. While rice cooks, steam broccoli florets in a steamer basket over boiling water for 4–5 minutes until bright green and just tender. Set aside.
3. In a small bowl, whisk together miso paste, maple syrup, rice vinegar, tamari, sesame oil, ginger, garlic, and black pepper until smooth.
4. Heat 2 teaspoons avocado oil in a large nonstick skillet over medium heat. Add tempeh cubes and cook for 3–4 minutes per side, turning to brown all surfaces.
5. Pour miso glaze over tempeh in the skillet. Toss to coat and cook for 2–3 minutes, stirring gently, until glaze thickens and tempeh is well coated. Remove from heat.
6. In the same skillet, add remaining 1 teaspoon avocado oil and steamed broccoli. Sauté for 1–2 minutes to heat through and lightly coat with any remaining glaze.
7. To assemble, divide brown rice between two bowls. Top each with glazed tempeh, broccoli, avocado slices, sesame seeds, and scallions. Serve warm.

Estimated total time

Prep time: 15 minutes
Cook time: 25 minutes
Total: 40 minutes

Nutritional facts per serving

Calories: 420
Protein: 22 g
Fat: 17 g
Carbs: 48 g
Fiber: 8 g
Sugar: 7 g

Dietary labels/tags

Gluten-free
Dairy-free
Vegan
Anti-inflammatory
Soy-free option
Low-glycemic

Suggested cooking method/program

Stovetop (rice, tempeh, broccoli)

Storage & meal prep tips

Store assembled bowls in airtight containers in the refrigerator for up to 3 days
Reheat gently in a skillet or microwave before serving
Avocado is best added fresh just before eating
Not recommended for freezing

Cortisol reset tip

Miso and tempeh provide fermented, gut-supportive probiotics and plant protein, while broccoli delivers sulforaphane to help lower inflammation and support hormone balance.

Possible variations

Add 1/2 cup (80 g) shredded carrots or red cabbage for extra color and crunch
Top with a drizzle of sriracha or chili crisp for gentle heat
Swap brown rice for millet or wild rice for variety
Use roasted Brussels sprouts or asparagus instead of broccoli
Add a handful of baby spinach to wilt into the bowl just before serving

44. Black Bean Avocado & Mango Salad with Lime-Ginger Dressing

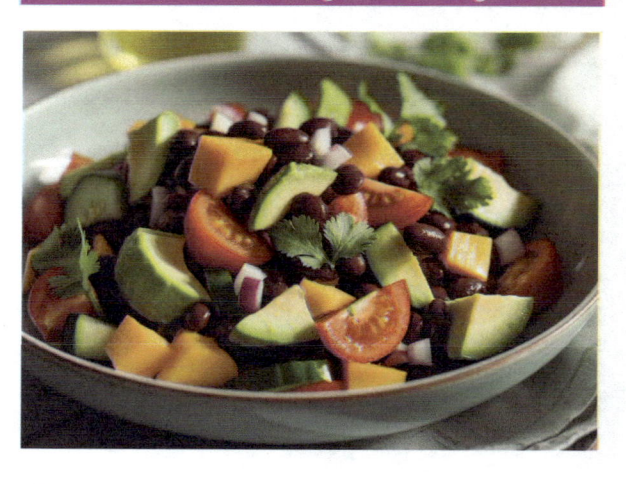

servings: 4

Ingredients

- 1 (15 oz/425 g) can no-salt-added black beans, drained and rinsed
- 1 cup (165 g) ripe mango, diced (about 1 medium)
- 1 cup (150 g) cherry tomatoes, quartered
- 1/2 cup (75 g) red bell pepper, diced
- 1/2 cup (75 g) English cucumber, diced
- 1/4 cup (30 g) red onion, finely diced
- 1 large ripe avocado, diced
- 1/4 cup (10 g) fresh cilantro, chopped
- 2 tablespoons (30 ml) extra-virgin olive oil
- 2 tablespoons (30 ml) fresh lime juice
- 1 tablespoon (15 ml) pure maple syrup
- 1 teaspoon (5 ml) grated fresh ginger
- 1/2 teaspoon (2 g) fine sea salt
- 1/4 teaspoon (0.5 g) ground black pepper
- Optional swaps: Use pineapple or papaya instead of mango; swap cilantro for fresh mint; omit onion for low-FODMAP; use lemon juice instead of lime

Directions

1. In a large mixing bowl, combine black beans, diced mango, cherry tomatoes, red bell pepper, cucumber, red onion, and cilantro.
2. In a small bowl or jar, whisk together olive oil, lime juice, maple syrup, grated ginger, sea salt, and black pepper until well emulsified.
3. Pour the dressing over the salad ingredients and toss gently to combine.
4. Add diced avocado and fold in carefully to avoid mashing.
5. Taste and adjust seasoning if needed.
6. Serve immediately, or chill for up to 1 hour for enhanced flavor.

Estimated total time

Prep time: 15 minutes
Cook time: 0 minutes
Total: 15 minutes

Nutritional facts per serving

Calories: 260
Protein: 7 g
Fat: 12 g
Carbs: 34 g
Fiber: 10 g
Sugar: 10 g

Dietary labels/tags

Gluten-free
Dairy-free
Vegan
Anti-inflammatory
Low-glycemic
Nut-free
Soy-free

Suggested cooking method/program

No-cook assembly

Storage & meal prep tips

Store in an airtight container in the refrigerator for up to 2 days
Best enjoyed fresh due to avocado; add avocado just before serving if prepping ahead
Not recommended for freezing

Cortisol reset tip

Black beans and avocado provide magnesium and fiber to help regulate blood sugar and support adrenal health, while mango and lime offer vitamin C and antioxidants to reduce inflammation.

Possible variations

Add 1/2 cup (80 g) cooked quinoa for extra protein and fiber
Top with 1/4 cup (30 g) toasted pumpkin seeds for crunch
Swap mango for diced peaches or nectarines in summer
Add 1/2 jalapeño, finely diced, for gentle heat
Serve over baby spinach or arugula for a heartier salad

HEARTY SOUPS & STEWS (5 RECIPES)

45. Turmeric Lentil & Sweet Potato Soup

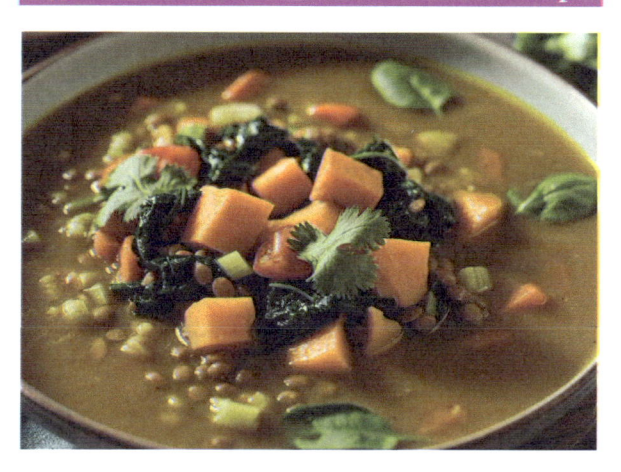

servings: 4

Ingredients

- 1 tablespoon (15 ml) extra-virgin olive oil
- 1 medium yellow onion, diced (about 1 cup/140 g)
- 2 medium carrots, peeled and diced (about 1 cup/130 g)
- 2 celery stalks, diced (about 3/4 cup/90 g)
- 3 cloves garlic, minced
- 1 tablespoon (6 g) fresh ginger, grated
- 1 1/2 teaspoons (4 g) ground turmeric
- 1 teaspoon (2 g) ground cumin
- 1/2 teaspoon (1 g) ground coriander
- 1/2 teaspoon (1 g) smoked paprika
- 1/4 teaspoon (0.5 g) ground black pepper
- 1 1/4 teaspoons (6 g) fine sea salt, divided
- 1 large sweet potato, peeled and diced (about 2 cups/300 g)
- 1 cup (200 g) dried red lentils, rinsed
- 5 cups (1.2 L) low-sodium vegetable broth
- 1 (14.5 oz/410 g) can no-salt-added diced tomatoes, with juices
- 2 cups (60 g) baby spinach, roughly chopped
- 1 tablespoon (15 ml) fresh lemon juice
- 1/4 cup (10 g) fresh cilantro, chopped, plus more for garnish
- Optional swaps: Use butternut squash instead of sweet potato; swap spinach for kale or chard; use green lentils (increase cook time by 10 minutes); omit onion and garlic for low-FODMAP; use avocado oil for higher smoke point

Directions

1. Heat olive oil in a large soup pot or Dutch oven over medium heat.
2. Add onion, carrots, and celery. Sauté for 5–6 minutes, stirring occasionally, until vegetables are softened.
3. Stir in garlic, ginger, turmeric, cumin, coriander, smoked paprika, black pepper, and 1 teaspoon salt. Cook for 1 minute until fragrant.
4. Add diced sweet potato and rinsed lentils. Stir to coat with spices.
5. Pour in vegetable broth and diced tomatoes with their juices. Bring to a boil over high heat.
6. Reduce heat to low, cover, and simmer for 20–22 minutes, stirring occasionally, until lentils and sweet potatoes are tender.
7. Stir in chopped spinach and cook for 2–3 minutes until wilted.
8. Remove from heat. Stir in lemon juice, cilantro, and remaining 1/4 teaspoon salt.
9. Taste and adjust seasoning as needed.
10. Ladle into bowls and garnish with extra cilantro if desired.

Estimated total time

Prep time: 15 minutes
Cook time: 30 minutes
Total: 45 minutes

Nutritional facts per serving

Calories: 260
Protein: 11 g
Fat: 5 g
Carbs: 45 g
Fiber: 11 g
Sugar: 9 g

Dietary labels/tags

Gluten-free
Dairy-free
Vegan
Anti-inflammatory
Nut-free
Soy-free
Low-glycemic

Suggested cooking method/program

Stovetop (large soup pot or Dutch oven)

Storage & meal prep tips

Store cooled soup in airtight containers in the refrigerator for up to 4 days
Freeze in individual portions for up to 2 months
Reheat gently on the stovetop or in the microwave, adding a splash of broth if needed to thin

Cortisol reset tip

Turmeric and ginger provide potent anti-inflammatory compounds, while lentils and sweet potatoes offer steady energy and fiber to help stabilize blood sugar and support adrenal balance.

Possible variations

Add 1/2 cup (80 g) frozen peas or corn in the last 5 minutes of cooking
Top with a dollop of unsweetened coconut yogurt for creaminess
Stir in 1/2 teaspoon red pepper flakes for gentle heat
Serve with a squeeze of fresh lime juice for extra brightness
Swap cilantro for fresh parsley if preferred

46. Ginger-Carrot Orange Immune Broth

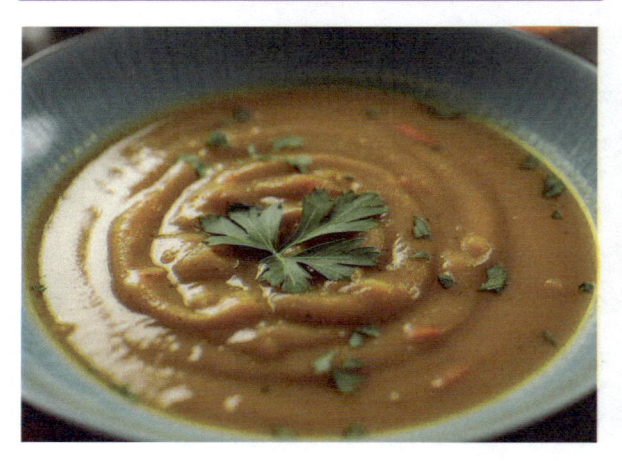

servings: 4

Ingredients

- 1 tablespoon (15 ml) extra-virgin olive oil
- 1 medium yellow onion, diced (about 1 cup/140 g)
- 3 large carrots, peeled and sliced (about 2 cups/260 g)
- 2 celery stalks, diced (about 3/4 cup/90 g)
- 1 tablespoon (15 g) fresh ginger, peeled and grated
- 2 cloves garlic, minced
- 1/2 teaspoon (1 g) ground turmeric
- 1/2 teaspoon (1 g) ground cumin
- 1/2 teaspoon (2 g) fine sea salt
- 1/4 teaspoon (0.5 g) ground black pepper

- 4 cups (950 ml) low-sodium vegetable broth
- 1 cup (240 ml) freshly squeezed orange juice (from about 2 large oranges)
- 1 tablespoon (15 ml) fresh lemon juice
- 1/4 cup (10 g) fresh parsley, chopped, plus more for garnish
- Optional swaps: Use avocado oil instead of olive oil; swap parsley for cilantro; omit onion and garlic for low-FODMAP; use bottled 100% orange juice if fresh is unavailable

Directions

1. Heat olive oil in a large saucepan or Dutch oven over medium heat
2. Add onion, carrots, and celery. Sauté for 5–6 minutes, stirring occasionally, until vegetables begin to soften
3. Stir in ginger, garlic, turmeric, cumin, salt, and black pepper. Cook for 1 minute until fragrant
4. Pour in vegetable broth and bring to a gentle boil
5. Reduce heat to low, cover, and simmer for 15–18 minutes, until carrots are very tender
6. Remove from heat. Stir in orange juice, lemon juice, and chopped parsley
7. Use an immersion blender to blend the soup directly in the pot until smooth, or transfer in batches to a blender (vent lid slightly) and blend until creamy
8. Taste and adjust seasoning if needed
9. Ladle into bowls and garnish with extra parsley if desired

Estimated total time

Prep time: 10 minutes
Cook time: 25 minutes
Total: 35 minutes

Nutritional facts per serving

Calories: 110
Protein: 2 g
Fat: 4 g
Carbs: 19 g
Fiber: 3 g
Sugar: 10 g

Dietary labels/tags

Gluten-free
Dairy-free
Vegan
Anti-inflammatory
Nut-free
Soy-free
Low-glycemic

Suggested cooking method/program

Stovetop (large saucepan or Dutch oven)

Storage & meal prep tips

Store cooled broth in airtight containers in the refrigerator for up to 4 days
Freeze in individual portions for up to 2 months
Reheat gently on the stovetop or in the microwave, stirring well before serving

Cortisol reset tip

Ginger and turmeric provide anti-inflammatory support, while vitamin C from orange juice helps modulate stress hormones and support immune resilience.

Possible variations

Add 1/2 cup (80 g) cooked red lentils for extra protein and fiber
Stir in 1/2 teaspoon ground coriander for a flavor twist
Top with a swirl of unsweetened coconut yogurt for creaminess
Add 1 cup (30 g) baby spinach in the last 2 minutes of cooking for extra greens
Swap orange juice for carrot juice for a deeper carrot flavor

47. Miso Mushroom & Baby Bok Choy Detox Soup

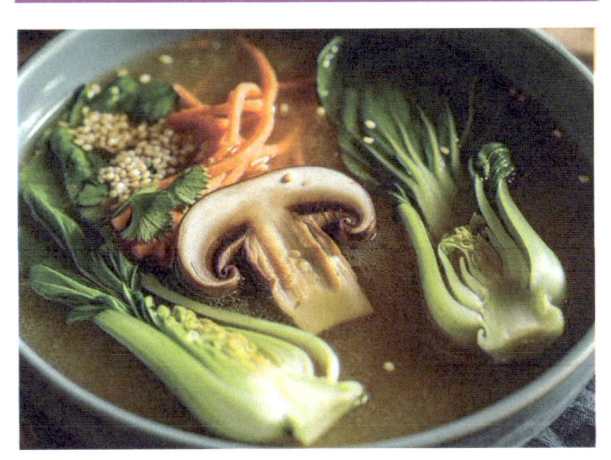

servings: 4

Ingredients

- 1 tablespoon (15 ml) avocado oil
- 1 medium yellow onion, diced (about 1 cup/140 g)
- 2 cloves garlic, minced

- 1 tablespoon (6 g) fresh ginger, peeled and grated
- 8 ounces (225 g) cremini or shiitake mushrooms, cleaned and sliced
- 4 cups (950 ml) low-sodium vegetable broth
- 2 cups (480 ml) filtered water
- 2 tablespoons (30 ml) coconut aminos
- 1 tablespoon (15 ml) rice vinegar
- 1/2 teaspoon (2 g) fine sea salt
- 1/4 teaspoon (0.5 g) ground black pepper
- 4 heads baby bok choy, ends trimmed and leaves separated (about 10 oz/280 g)
- 1/2 cup (30 g) shredded carrots
- 3 tablespoons (45 g) white or yellow miso paste
- 1/4 cup (10 g) fresh cilantro, chopped, plus more for garnish
- 1 tablespoon (10 g) toasted sesame seeds, for garnish
- Optional swaps: Use tamari instead of coconut aminos for gluten-free; swap cremini for button mushrooms; omit onion and garlic for low-FODMAP; use spinach instead of bok choy

Directions

1. Heat avocado oil in a large soup pot over medium heat
2. Add diced onion and sauté for 3–4 minutes, stirring occasionally, until translucent
3. Stir in garlic and ginger, cooking for 1 minute until fragrant
4. Add sliced mushrooms and cook for 4–5 minutes, stirring, until softened and lightly browned
5. Pour in vegetable broth and filtered water
6. Stir in coconut aminos, rice vinegar, sea salt, and black pepper
7. Bring to a gentle boil, then reduce heat to low and simmer for 8 minutes
8. Add baby bok choy and shredded carrots, simmering for 3–4 minutes until bok choy is just tender
9. In a small bowl, whisk miso paste with 1/2 cup (120 ml) hot soup broth until smooth
10. Stir miso mixture back into the pot (do not boil after adding miso to preserve probiotics)
11. Remove from heat, stir in chopped cilantro
12. Taste and adjust seasoning if needed
13. Ladle into bowls and garnish with extra cilantro and toasted sesame seeds

Estimated total time

Prep time: 10 minutes
Cook time: 20 minutes
Total: 30 minutes

Nutritional facts per serving

Calories: 90
Protein: 4 g
Fat: 4 g
Carbs: 12 g
Fiber: 3 g
Sugar: 4 g

Dietary labels/tags

Gluten-free
Dairy-free
Vegan
Anti-inflammatory
Nut-free
Soy-free (if using coconut aminos)
Low-glycemic

Suggested cooking method/program

Stovetop (large soup pot)

Storage & meal prep tips

Store cooled soup in airtight containers in the refrigerator for up to 3 days
Reheat gently on the stovetop over low heat; do not boil after adding miso
Freeze without miso for up to 1 month; stir in fresh miso after reheating

Cortisol reset tip

Miso provides gut-friendly probiotics, while mushrooms and bok choy deliver antioxidants and adaptogenic support to help modulate stress and inflammation.

Possible variations

Add 1/2 cup (80 g) cooked brown rice or quinoa for a heartier meal
Stir in 1 cup (30 g) baby spinach in the last minute of cooking
Top with a drizzle of chili oil for gentle heat
Swap cilantro for fresh basil or parsley

48. Mediterranean White Bean Stew with Kale & Olives

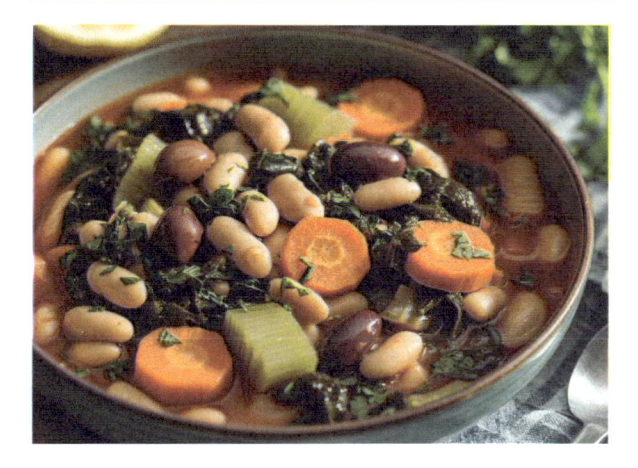

servings: 4

Ingredients

- 1 tablespoon (15 ml) extra-virgin olive oil
- 1 medium yellow onion, diced (about 1 cup/140 g)
- 2 cloves garlic, minced
- 2 medium carrots, peeled and sliced (about 1 cup/130 g)
- 2 celery stalks, diced (about 3/4 cup/90 g)
- 1 teaspoon (2 g) dried oregano
- 1/2 teaspoon (1 g) smoked paprika
- 1/2 teaspoon (2 g) fine sea salt
- 1/4 teaspoon (0.5 g) ground black pepper
- 1 (15-ounce/425 g) can no-salt-added diced tomatoes, with juices
- 2 (15-ounce/425 g each) cans no-salt-added white beans (cannellini or great northern), drained and rinsed
- 3 cups (710 ml) low-sodium vegetable broth
- 1 small bunch lacinato kale, stems removed and leaves chopped (about 4 cups/120 g)
- 1/2 cup (70 g) pitted Kalamata olives, halved
- 2 tablespoons (8 g) fresh parsley, chopped, plus more for garnish
- 1 tablespoon (15 ml) fresh lemon juice
- Optional swaps: Use avocado oil instead of olive oil; swap kale for baby spinach; omit onion and garlic for low-FODMAP; use green olives instead of Kalamata

Directions

1. Heat olive oil in a large Dutch oven or soup pot over medium heat
2. Add diced onion, carrots, and celery. Sauté for 5–6 minutes, stirring occasionally, until vegetables are softened
3. Stir in garlic, oregano, smoked paprika, salt, and black pepper. Cook for 1 minute until fragrant
4. Add diced tomatoes (with juices), white beans, and vegetable broth. Stir to combine
5. Bring to a gentle boil, then reduce heat to low and simmer uncovered for 12–15 minutes, until vegetables are tender and flavors meld
6. Stir in chopped kale and olives. Simmer for 3–4 minutes, until kale is wilted but still vibrant
7. Remove from heat. Stir in parsley and lemon juice
8. Taste and adjust seasoning if needed
9. Ladle into bowls and garnish with extra parsley if desired

Estimated total time

Prep time: 10 minutes
Cook time: 25 minutes
Total: 35 minutes

Nutritional facts per serving

Calories: 230
Protein: 9 g
Fat: 7 g
Carbs: 34 g
Fiber: 9 g
Sugar: 5 g

Dietary labels/tags

Gluten-free
Dairy-free
Vegan
Anti-inflammatory
Nut-free
Soy-free
Low-glycemic

Suggested cooking method/program

Stovetop (large Dutch oven or soup pot)

Storage & meal prep tips

Store cooled stew in airtight containers in the refrigerator for up to 4 days
Freeze in individual portions for up to 2 months
Reheat gently on the stovetop, adding a splash of broth or water if needed

Cortisol reset tip

White beans and kale provide magnesium and fiber to support balanced blood sugar and stress resilience, while olives offer healthy fats and polyphenols for anti-inflammatory benefits.

Possible variations

Add 1/2 cup (80 g) cooked quinoa for extra protein and texture
Stir in 1/2 teaspoon crushed red pepper for gentle heat
Top with a spoonful of unsweetened coconut yogurt for creaminess
Swap parsley for fresh basil or dill
Add 1/2 cup (80 g) artichoke hearts for a Mediterranean twist

49. Coconut Curry Chickpea & Spinach Stew

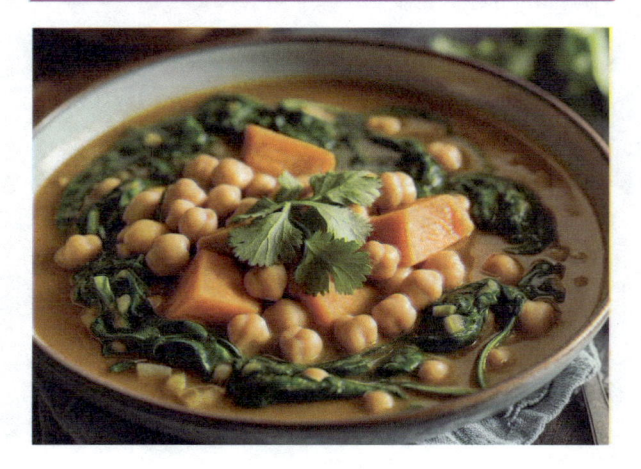

servings: 4

Ingredients

- 1 tablespoon (15 ml) avocado oil
- 1 medium yellow onion, diced (about 1 cup/140 g)
- 2 cloves garlic, minced
- 1 tablespoon (6 g) fresh ginger, peeled and grated
- 1 tablespoon (6 g) mild curry powder
- 1/2 teaspoon (2 g) ground turmeric
- 1/2 teaspoon (2 g) fine sea salt
- 1/4 teaspoon (0.5 g) ground black pepper
- 1 (15-ounce/425 g) can no-salt-added chickpeas, drained and rinsed
- 1 (14-ounce/400 ml) can full-fat coconut milk
- 1 cup (240 ml) low-sodium vegetable broth
- 1 medium sweet potato, peeled and diced (about 1 1/2 cups/200 g)
- 4 cups (120 g) baby spinach, packed
- 1 tablespoon (15 ml) fresh lime juice
- 2 tablespoons (8 g) fresh cilantro, chopped, plus more for garnish
- Optional swaps: Use olive oil instead of avocado oil; swap sweet potato for butternut squash; use kale instead of spinach; omit onion and garlic for low-FODMAP; use light coconut milk for lower fat

Directions

1. Heat avocado oil in a large Dutch oven or soup pot over medium heat
2. Add diced onion and sauté for 3–4 minutes, stirring occasionally, until translucent
3. Stir in garlic and ginger, cooking for 1 minute until fragrant
4. Sprinkle in curry powder, turmeric, sea salt, and black pepper; stir for 30 seconds to bloom spices
5. Add chickpeas, coconut milk, vegetable broth, and diced sweet potato
6. Stir well, bring to a gentle boil, then reduce heat to low
7. Cover and simmer for 15–18 minutes, until sweet potato is fork-tender
8. Uncover, add baby spinach, and cook for 2–3 minutes, stirring, until wilted
9. Remove from heat, stir in lime juice and chopped cilantro
10. Taste and adjust seasoning if needed
11. Ladle into bowls and garnish with extra cilantro

Estimated total time

Prep time: 10 minutes
Cook time: 25 minutes
Total: 35 minutes

Nutritional facts per serving

Calories: 320
Protein: 8 g
Fat: 17 g
Carbs: 36 g
Fiber: 8 g
Sugar: 7 g

Dietary labels/tags

Gluten-free
Dairy-free
Vegan
Anti-inflammatory
Nut-free
Soy-free
Low-glycemic

Suggested cooking method/program

Stovetop (large Dutch oven or soup pot)

Storage & meal prep tips

Store cooled stew in airtight containers in the refrigerator for up to 4 days
Freeze in individual portions for up to 2 months

Reheat gently on the stovetop, adding a splash of broth or water if needed

Cortisol reset tip

Chickpeas and spinach provide magnesium and B vitamins to support adrenal health, while coconut milk and turmeric offer anti-inflammatory fats and phytonutrients to help balance stress hormones.

Possible variations

Add 1/2 cup (80 g) cooked brown rice or quinoa for extra heartiness
Stir in 1/2 teaspoon crushed red pepper for gentle heat
Top with a spoonful of unsweetened coconut yogurt for creaminess
Swap cilantro for fresh basil or parsley
Add 1/2 cup (80 g) diced red bell pepper with the sweet potato for extra color and vitamin C

PROTEIN-PACKED WRAPS & PLATES

50. Turmeric-Grilled Turkey, Avocado & Spinach Wrap

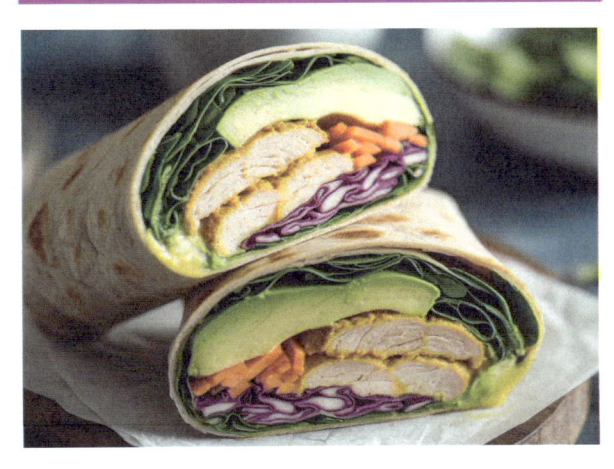

servings: 2

Ingredients

- 2 (4-ounce/115 g each) turkey breast cutlets
- 1 tablespoon (15 ml) avocado oil
- 1 teaspoon (2 g) ground turmeric
- 1/2 teaspoon (1 g) ground cumin
- 1/2 teaspoon (2 g) fine sea salt
- 1/4 teaspoon (0.5 g) ground black pepper
- 2 large gluten-free wraps or whole-grain tortillas (about 9-inch/23 cm each)
- 1 small ripe avocado, sliced (about 1/2 cup/75 g)
- 2 cups (60 g) baby spinach, packed
- 1/2 cup (60 g) shredded purple cabbage
- 1/4 cup (30 g) shredded carrots
- 2 tablespoons (30 ml) fresh lemon juice
- Optional swaps: Use grilled chicken breast instead of turkey; swap spinach for arugula; use collard green leaves for a grain-free wrap; omit cabbage for low-FODMAP

Directions

1. Pat turkey cutlets dry with paper towels.
2. In a small bowl, mix avocado oil, turmeric, cumin, sea salt, and black pepper.
3. Brush both sides of turkey cutlets with the spice oil mixture.
4. Preheat a grill pan or outdoor grill to medium-high heat.
5. Grill turkey cutlets for 3–4 minutes per side, or until cooked through and internal temperature reaches 165°F (74°C).
6. Transfer turkey to a cutting board and let rest for 2 minutes, then slice thinly.
7. Warm wraps or tortillas in a dry skillet for 20–30 seconds per side to make them pliable.
8. Lay wraps flat. Arrange spinach, cabbage, carrots, and avocado slices evenly down the center of each wrap.
9. Top with sliced grilled turkey.
10. Drizzle with fresh lemon juice.
11. Roll up tightly, tucking in the sides as you go. Slice in half to serve.

Estimated total time

Prep time: 10 minutes
Cook time: 10 minutes
Total: 20 minutes

Nutritional facts per serving

Calories: 340
Protein: 29 g
Fat: 15 g
Carbs: 28 g
Fiber: 7 g
Sugar: 3 g

Dietary labels/tags

Gluten-free (with GF wraps)
Dairy-free
Anti-inflammatory
High-protein
Soy-free
Low-glycemic

Suggested cooking method/program

Grill pan or outdoor grill

Storage & meal prep tips

Wraps can be assembled up to 1 day ahead; store tightly wrapped in the refrigerator
For best texture, add avocado just before serving
Grilled turkey can be cooked in advance and refrigerated for up to 3 days

Cortisol reset tip

Turkey provides lean protein to stabilize blood sugar and support muscle repair, while turmeric and avocado deliver anti-inflammatory compounds and healthy fats to help modulate stress hormones.

Possible variations

Add 2 tablespoons (30 g) hummus or dairy-free yogurt for extra creaminess
Swap turkey for grilled tempeh or tofu for a plant-based option
Include thinly sliced cucumber or bell pepper for extra crunch
Use a collard green leaf as a wrap for a grain-free, low-carb version
Sprinkle with hemp seeds or pumpkin seeds for added magnesium and texture

51. Lemon-Dill Tuna & Cannellini Bean Plate with Arugula

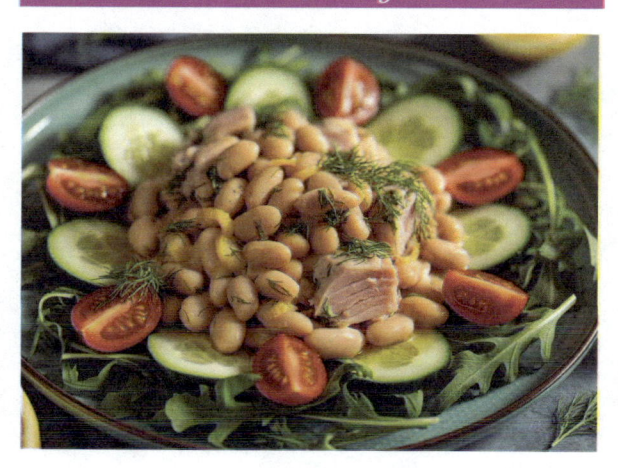

servings: 2

Ingredients

- 1 (5-ounce / 142 g) can wild-caught tuna in water, drained
- 1 cup (170 g) canned no-salt-added cannellini beans, drained and rinsed
- 2 cups (60 g) baby arugula, packed
- 1/2 cup (75 g) cherry tomatoes, halved
- 1/4 cup (30 g) thinly sliced cucumber
- 2 tablespoons (8 g) fresh dill, chopped
- 2 tablespoons (30 ml) extra-virgin olive oil
- 2 tablespoons (30 ml) fresh lemon juice
- 1 teaspoon (2 g) lemon zest
- 1/2 teaspoon (2 g) fine sea salt
- 1/4 teaspoon (0.5 g) ground black pepper
- Optional swaps: Use canned salmon instead of tuna; swap arugula for baby spinach; use white beans or navy beans instead of cannellini; omit tomatoes for low-FODMAP

Directions

1. In a medium bowl, combine drained tuna, cannellini beans, chopped dill, 1 tablespoon (15 ml) olive oil, 1 tablespoon (15 ml) lemon juice, lemon zest, 1/4 teaspoon (1 g) sea salt, and 1/8 teaspoon (0.25 g) black pepper
2. Gently toss with a fork to combine, breaking up tuna slightly but leaving some chunks
3. In a separate bowl, toss arugula, cherry tomatoes, and cucumber with remaining 1 tablespoon (15 ml) olive oil, 1 tablespoon (15 ml) lemon juice, 1/4 teaspoon (1 g) sea salt, and 1/8 teaspoon (0.25 g) black pepper
4. Divide arugula mixture evenly between two plates
5. Top each plate with half the tuna and bean mixture
6. Serve immediately, garnished with extra dill if desired

Estimated total time

Prep time: 10 minutes
Cook time: 0 minutes
Total: 10 minutes

Nutritional facts per serving

Calories: 320
Protein: 23 g
Fat: 14 g
Carbs: 27 g
Fiber: 7 g
Sugar: 3 g

Dietary labels/tags

Gluten-free
Dairy-free
Anti-inflammatory
High-protein
Soy-free
Low-glycemic

Suggested cooking method/program

No-cook (assembly only)

Storage & meal prep tips

Store assembled tuna and bean mixture in an airtight container in the refrigerator for up to 2 days
Keep arugula and vegetables separate until ready to serve for best texture
Add dressing just before serving to prevent sogginess

Cortisol reset tip

Tuna and cannellini beans provide lean protein and magnesium to help stabilize blood sugar and support adrenal function, while olive oil and dill offer anti-inflammatory benefits to help modulate stress response

Possible variations

Add 1/4 cup (35 g) sliced Kalamata olives for Mediterranean flavor
Top with 1 tablespoon (10 g) toasted pumpkin seeds for extra crunch and magnesium
Swap dill for fresh basil or parsley
Include 1/4 cup (40 g) diced roasted red pepper for sweetness and color
Serve over cooked quinoa or brown rice for a heartier meal

52. Miso-Glazed Tempeh Lettuce Wraps with Ginger Slaw

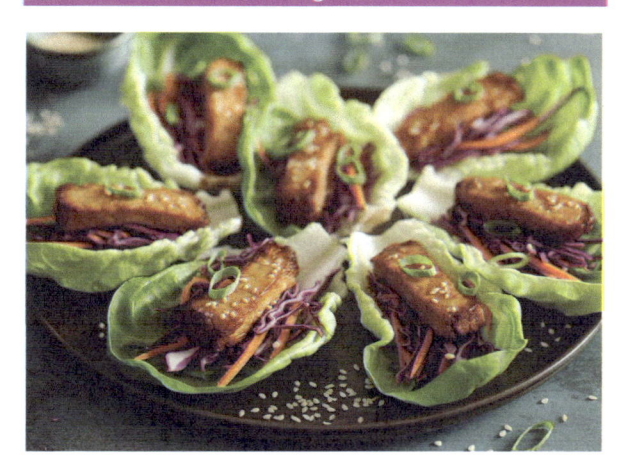

servings: 2

Ingredients

- 1 (8-ounce / 227 g) package organic tempeh, cut into 1/2-inch (1.25 cm) strips
- 2 tablespoons (30 ml) white or yellow miso paste
- 1 tablespoon (15 ml) pure maple syrup
- 1 tablespoon (15 ml) coconut aminos or low-sodium tamari
- 1 tablespoon (15 ml) rice vinegar
- 1 tablespoon (15 ml) avocado oil
- 1/2 teaspoon (2 g) grated fresh ginger
- 1/2 teaspoon (2 g) garlic powder
- 8 large butter lettuce leaves (about 60 g)
- 1 cup (70 g) shredded red cabbage
- 1/2 cup (60 g) shredded carrots
- 1/4 cup (30 g) thinly sliced scallions
- 2 tablespoons (30 ml) fresh lime juice
- 1 tablespoon (15 ml) toasted sesame oil
- 1 tablespoon (10 g) sesame seeds
- 1/4 teaspoon (1 g) fine sea salt
- Optional swaps: Use gluten-free tamari for gluten-free; swap tempeh for extra-firm tofu; use romaine leaves instead of butter lettuce; omit sesame seeds for nut/seed allergies

Directions

1. In a small bowl, whisk together miso paste, maple syrup, coconut aminos, rice vinegar, avocado oil, grated ginger, and garlic powder until smooth
2. Place tempeh strips in a shallow dish and pour miso glaze over, turning to coat all sides. Let marinate for 10 minutes
3. While tempeh marinates, combine shredded cabbage, carrots, scallions, lime juice, sesame oil, sesame seeds, and sea salt in a medium bowl. Toss well to combine and set aside
4. Heat a large nonstick skillet over medium heat. Add marinated tempeh strips in a single layer (reserve extra marinade)
5. Cook tempeh for 3–4 minutes per side, brushing with reserved marinade, until golden and caramelized
6. Remove tempeh from skillet and let cool slightly
7. Lay out butter lettuce leaves. Divide ginger slaw evenly among leaves
8. Top each with 2–3 strips of miso-glazed tempeh
9. Serve immediately, garnished with extra scallions or sesame seeds if desired

Estimated total time

Prep time: 15 minutes
Cook time: 10 minutes
Total: 25 minutes

Nutritional facts per serving

Calories: 320
Protein: 19 g
Fat: 15 g
Carbs: 28 g
Fiber: 7 g
Sugar: 8 g

Dietary labels/tags

Gluten-free (with GF tamari)
Dairy-free
Vegan
Anti-inflammatory
Soy-based - Low-glycemic

Suggested cooking method/program

Nonstick skillet (stovetop)

Storage & meal prep tips

Store cooked tempeh and slaw separately in airtight containers in the refrigerator for up to 3 days
Assemble wraps just before serving for best texture
Tempeh can be reheated in a skillet or microwave

Cortisol reset tip

Tempeh offers plant-based protein and gut-friendly probiotics, while miso and ginger provide anti-inflammatory benefits to help balance stress hormones and support digestion

Possible variations

Add 1/4 cup (35 g) diced mango or pineapple to the slaw for a sweet-tart twist
Swap tempeh for grilled chicken or shrimp for an omnivore option
Include thinly sliced cucumber or bell pepper for extra crunch
Top with fresh cilantro or mint for added freshness
Serve with a side of brown rice or quinoa for a more filling meal

53. Warm Quinoa, Roasted Chickpea & Walnut Power Plate

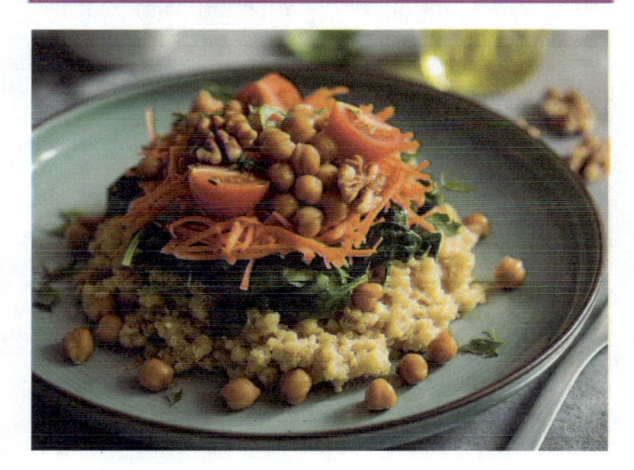

servings: 2

Ingredients

- 1/2 cup (90 g) dry quinoa, rinsed
- 1 cup (240 ml) low-sodium vegetable broth or water
- 1 (15-ounce / 425 g) can no-salt-added chickpeas, drained and rinsed
- 1 tablespoon (15 ml) avocado oil
- 1 teaspoon (2 g) smoked paprika
- 1/2 teaspoon (1 g) ground cumin
- 1/2 teaspoon (2 g) fine sea salt
- 1/4 teaspoon (0.5 g) ground black pepper
- 2 cups (60 g) baby spinach, packed
- 1/2 cup (60 g) shredded carrots
- 1/2 cup (75 g) cherry tomatoes, halved
- 1/4 cup (30 g) raw walnuts, roughly chopped
- 2 tablespoons (30 ml) extra-virgin olive oil
- 2 tablespoons (30 ml) fresh lemon juice
- 1 tablespoon (4 g) fresh parsley, chopped
- Optional swaps: Use brown rice or millet instead of quinoa; swap walnuts for pecans or pumpkin seeds; use kale or arugula instead of spinach; omit walnuts for nut-free

Directions

1. Preheat oven to 400°F (205°C). Line a baking sheet with parchment paper
2. Pat chickpeas dry with a clean towel. In a bowl, toss chickpeas with avocado oil, smoked paprika, cumin, 1/4 teaspoon (1 g) sea salt, and black pepper
3. Spread chickpeas in a single layer on prepared baking sheet. Roast for 20–25 minutes, shaking halfway, until golden and crisp
4. While chickpeas roast, combine quinoa and vegetable broth in a small saucepan. Bring to a boil, reduce heat to low, cover, and simmer for 15 minutes until liquid is absorbed. Remove from heat and let stand, covered, for 5 minutes. Fluff with a fork
5. In a large bowl, toss baby spinach, shredded carrots, and cherry tomatoes with olive oil, lemon juice, remaining 1/4 teaspoon (1 g) sea salt, and parsley
6. Divide quinoa between two plates. Top each with half the spinach mixture, roasted chickpeas, and chopped walnuts
7. Serve warm, garnished with extra parsley if desired

Estimated total time

Prep time: 10 minutes
Cook time: 25 minutes
Total: 35 minutes

Nutritional facts per serving

Calories: 410
Protein: 13 g
Fat: 22 g
Carbs: 44 g
Fiber: 9 g
Sugar: 5 g

Dietary labels/tags

Gluten-free
Dairy-free
Vegan
Anti-inflammatory
High-fiber
Soy-free

Suggested cooking method/program

Oven roasting (for chickpeas)
Stovetop (for quinoa)

Storage & meal prep tips

Store components separately in airtight containers in the refrigerator for up to 3 days
Reheat quinoa and chickpeas before assembling for best texture
Add fresh greens just before serving to maintain crispness

Cortisol reset tip

Quinoa and walnuts provide magnesium and plant-based protein to help regulate cortisol, while roasted chickpeas and leafy greens offer fiber and antioxidants to reduce inflammation

Possible variations

Add 1/4 cup (35 g) diced roasted sweet potato for extra sweetness
Top with 1 tablespoon (10 g) hemp seeds for added omega-3s
Swap smoked paprika for curry powder for a different flavor profile
Include 1/4 avocado, sliced, for healthy fats and creaminess. Serve with a dollop of plain unsweetened coconut yogurt for a tangy finish

54. Harissa-Lime Grilled Salmon with Zucchini Ribbons

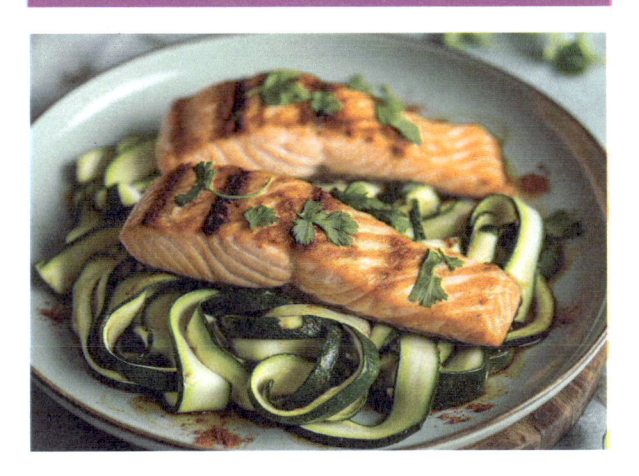

servings: 2

Ingredients

- 2 (5-ounce / 140 g each) wild-caught salmon fillets, skin on
- 1 tablespoon (15 ml) harissa paste
- 1 tablespoon (15 ml) extra-virgin olive oil
- 1 tablespoon (15 ml) fresh lime juice
- 1 teaspoon (2 g) lime zest
- 1/2 teaspoon (2 g) garlic powder
- 1/4 teaspoon (1 g) fine sea salt
- 1/4 teaspoon (0.5 g) ground black pepper
- 2 medium zucchini (about 12 ounces / 340 g total), ends trimmed
- 1 tablespoon (15 ml) extra-virgin olive oil (for zucchini)
- 1 tablespoon (15 ml) fresh chopped cilantro or parsley
- Optional swaps: Use mild chili paste instead of harissa for less heat; swap salmon for arctic char or steelhead trout; use yellow squash in place of zucchini; omit cilantro for cilantro sensitivity

Directions

1. In a small bowl, whisk together harissa paste, 1 tablespoon olive oil, lime juice, lime zest, garlic powder, sea salt, and black pepper
2. Pat salmon fillets dry with paper towels. Place in a shallow dish and brush all over with harissa-lime marinade. Let stand at room temperature for 10 minutes
3. While salmon marinates, use a vegetable peeler to shave zucchini into long, thin ribbons
4. Toss zucchini ribbons with 1 tablespoon olive oil and a pinch of sea salt in a medium bowl
5. Preheat a grill or grill pan over medium-high heat. Oil grates lightly

6. Place salmon fillets skin-side down on the grill. Cook for 4–5 minutes, then carefully flip and grill for another 3–4 minutes, or until salmon is just opaque and flakes easily with a fork
7. While salmon cooks, grill zucchini ribbons in a grill basket or directly on the grill for 1–2 minutes per side, just until tender and lightly charred
8. Transfer grilled zucchini to plates. Top each with a salmon fillet
9. Sprinkle with fresh cilantro or parsley before serving

Estimated total time

Prep time: 10 minutes
Cook time: 12 minutes
Total: 22 minutes

Nutritional facts per serving

Calories: 340
Protein: 30 g
Fat: 20 g
Carbs: 7 g
Fiber: 2 g
Sugar: 4 g

Dietary labels/tags

Gluten-free
Dairy-free
Paleo-friendly
Anti-inflammatory
Low-carb
Soy-free

Suggested cooking method/program

Outdoor grill or stovetop grill pan

Storage & meal prep tips

Store cooked salmon and zucchini separately in airtight containers in the refrigerator for up to 2 days
Reheat salmon gently in a skillet over low heat or enjoy cold over greens
Zucchini ribbons are best enjoyed fresh but can be eaten chilled

Cortisol reset tip

Wild salmon provides omega-3s to help lower inflammation and support hormone balance, while harissa and lime add antioxidants to help your body manage stress

Possible variations

Top with 1/4 avocado, sliced, for extra healthy fats

Add a handful of arugula or baby spinach under the zucchini for more greens
Swap harissa for a blend of smoked paprika and cumin for a milder flavor
Serve with a side of quinoa or brown rice for a more filling meal

5 LUNCHBOX RECIPES FOR BUSY DAYS

55. Herbed White Bean & Arugula Mason Jar Salad

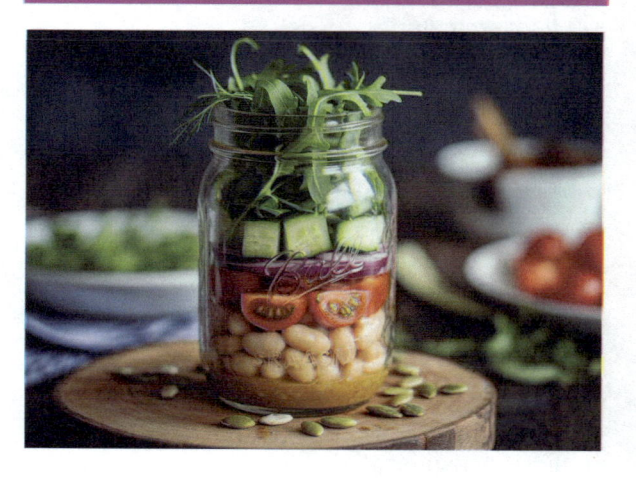

servings: 2

Ingredients

- 1 (15-ounce / 425 g) can no-salt-added cannellini beans, drained and rinsed
- 2 tablespoons (30 ml) extra-virgin olive oil
- 1 tablespoon (15 ml) apple cider vinegar
- 1 teaspoon (2 g) Dijon mustard
- 1/2 teaspoon (2 g) fine sea salt
- 1/4 teaspoon (0.5 g) ground black pepper
- 1/2 cup (75 g) cherry tomatoes, quartered
- 1/2 cup (60 g) cucumber, diced
- 1/4 cup (30 g) red onion, finely diced
- 1/4 cup (4 g) fresh parsley, chopped
- 1 tablespoon (2 g) fresh dill, chopped
- 2 cups (60 g) baby arugula, packed
- 1/4 cup (30 g) raw pumpkin seeds (pepitas)
- Optional swaps: Use navy beans or great northern beans instead of cannellini; swap arugula for baby spinach or mixed greens; omit onion for low-FODMAP; use sunflower seeds for nut-free

Directions

1. In a small bowl, whisk together olive oil, apple cider vinegar, Dijon mustard, sea salt, and black pepper until emulsified

2. Divide dressing evenly between two wide-mouth quart-size mason jars (about 1 tablespoon per jar)
3. Layer quartered cherry tomatoes, diced cucumber, and red onion over the dressing in each jar
4. Add half the cannellini beans to each jar, then sprinkle with chopped parsley and dill
5. Top each jar with 1 cup baby arugula and 2 tablespoons pumpkin seeds
6. Seal jars tightly and refrigerate until ready to eat
7. To serve, shake the jar to distribute the dressing, or pour contents into a bowl and toss

Estimated total time

Prep time: 12 minutes
No cook time
Total: 12 minutes

Nutritional facts per serving

Calories: 340
Protein: 13 g
Fat: 18 g
Carbs: 34 g
Fiber: 9 g
Sugar: 4 g

Dietary labels/tags

Gluten-free
Dairy-free
Vegan
Anti-inflammatory
High-fiber
Soy-free

Suggested cooking method/program

No-cook, mason jar assembly

Storage & meal prep tips

Store assembled salads in sealed mason jars in the refrigerator for up to 3 days
Keep upright to prevent greens from getting soggy
Shake or toss just before eating

Cortisol reset tip

Beans and pumpkin seeds provide magnesium and plant-based protein to help regulate cortisol, while arugula and fresh herbs offer antioxidants to reduce inflammation

Possible variations

Add 1/4 avocado, diced, for extra healthy fats
Swap pumpkin seeds for hemp hearts for more omega-3s
Include 1/4 cup (35 g) roasted sweet potato cubes for a heartier salad
Use lemon juice instead of apple cider vinegar for a brighter flavor
Add 2 tablespoons (20 g) crumbled feta if dairy is tolerated

56. Warm Farro with Roasted Brussels Sprouts & Pomegranate

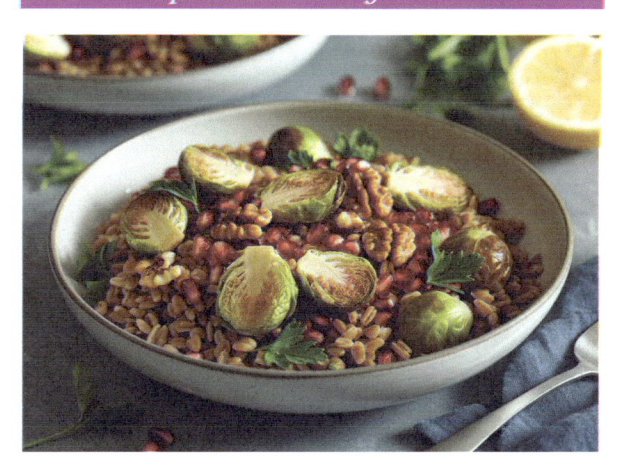

servings: 2

Ingredients

- 1/2 cup (90 g) uncooked farro, rinsed
- 1 cup (240 ml) low-sodium vegetable broth
- 8 ounces (225 g) Brussels sprouts, trimmed and halved
- 1 tablespoon (15 ml) extra-virgin olive oil
- 1/4 teaspoon (1 g) fine sea salt
- 1/4 teaspoon (0.5 g) ground black pepper
- 1/2 teaspoon (1 g) ground cumin
- 1/2 cup (80 g) pomegranate arils
- 2 tablespoons (20 g) toasted walnuts, chopped
- 2 tablespoons (8 g) fresh parsley, chopped
- 1 tablespoon (15 ml) fresh lemon juice
- Optional swaps: Use quinoa or brown rice for gluten-free; swap walnuts for pumpkin seeds for nut-free; use dried cranberries if pomegranate is unavailable

Directions

1. Preheat oven to 425°F (220°C). Line a baking sheet with parchment paper
2. Toss halved Brussels sprouts with olive oil, sea salt, black pepper, and cumin. Spread in a single layer on the prepared baking sheet
3. Roast Brussels sprouts for 20–22 minutes, stirring halfway, until golden and tender
4. While sprouts roast, combine farro and vegetable broth in a medium saucepan. Bring

to a boil, then reduce heat to low, cover, and simmer for 20 minutes, or until farro is tender and liquid is absorbed. Fluff with a fork
5. In a large bowl, combine cooked farro, roasted Brussels sprouts, pomegranate arils, toasted walnuts, and parsley
6. Drizzle with lemon juice and toss gently to combine
7. Divide between two bowls and serve warm

Estimated total time

Prep time: 10 minutes
Cook time: 25 minutes
Total: 35 minutes

Nutritional facts per serving

Calories: 340
Protein: 9 g
Fat: 14 g
Carbs: 48 g
Fiber: 9 g
Sugar: 10 g

Dietary labels/tags

Vegetarian
Dairy-free
Anti-inflammatory
High-fiber
Soy-free

Suggested cooking method/program

Oven roasting and stovetop simmer

Storage & meal prep tips

Store leftovers in an airtight container in the refrigerator for up to 3 days
Reheat gently in a skillet over medium-low heat, adding a splash of broth if needed

Cortisol reset tip

Farro and Brussels sprouts provide fiber and B vitamins to support steady energy and hormone balance, while pomegranate adds antioxidants to help reduce inflammation

Possible variations

Add 1/4 cup (35 g) crumbled feta if dairy is tolerated
Swap parsley for fresh mint for a brighter flavor
Top with 1/2 avocado, sliced, for extra healthy fats

57. Grilled Chicken, Avocado & Turmeric Slaw Wrap

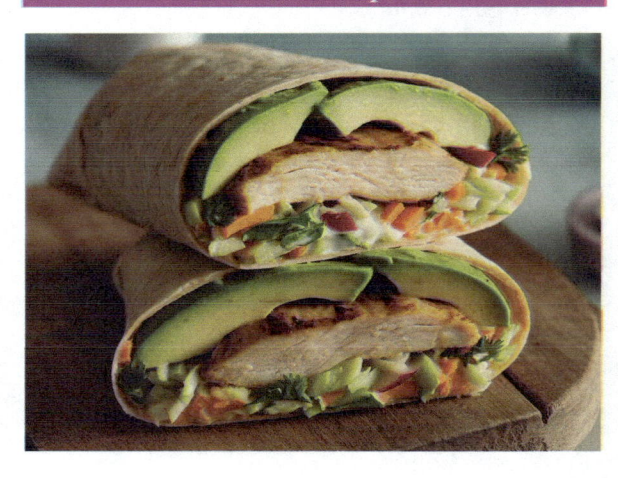

servings: 2

Ingredients

- 2 (4-ounce / 115 g each) boneless, skinless chicken breasts
- 1 tablespoon (15 ml) extra-virgin olive oil
- 1/2 teaspoon (1 g) ground turmeric
- 1/2 teaspoon (1 g) smoked paprika
- 1/2 teaspoon (2 g) fine sea salt
- 1/4 teaspoon (0.5 g) ground black pepper
- 1 cup (70 g) shredded green cabbage
- 1/2 cup (35 g) shredded carrots
- 1/4 cup (30 g) red bell pepper, thinly sliced
- 2 tablespoons (30 ml) plain unsweetened coconut yogurt
- 1 tablespoon (15 ml) apple cider vinegar
- 1 teaspoon (5 ml) honey or pure maple syrup
- 1/2 ripe avocado, sliced
- 2 large (8-inch / 20 cm) gluten-free or whole-grain wraps
- 2 tablespoons (8 g) fresh cilantro, chopped
- Optional swaps: Use tofu or tempeh for vegetarian; swap coconut yogurt for Greek yogurt if dairy is tolerated; use collard green leaves for grain-free/low-carb

Directions

1. Preheat a grill pan or outdoor grill to medium-high heat
2. In a small bowl, mix olive oil, turmeric, smoked paprika, sea salt, and black pepper
3. Brush chicken breasts with the spice oil mixture on both sides
4. Grill chicken for 4–5 minutes per side, or until cooked through and internal temperature reaches 165°F (74°C). Let rest 2 minutes, then slice thinly
5. In a medium bowl, combine shredded cabbage, carrots, red bell pepper, coconut

yogurt, apple cider vinegar, and honey. Toss well to coat
6. Warm wraps in a dry skillet for 30 seconds per side or until pliable
7. Lay wraps flat. Divide turmeric slaw between wraps, top with sliced grilled chicken, avocado, and cilantro
8. Roll up tightly, tucking in the sides as you go. Slice in half to serve

Estimated total time

Prep time: 15 minutes
Cook time: 10 minutes
Total: 25 minutes

Nutritional facts per serving

Calories: 370
Protein: 28 g
Fat: 15 g
Carbs: 32 g
Fiber: 7 g
Sugar: 7 g

Dietary labels/tags

Gluten-free (with GF wraps)
Dairy-free
Anti-inflammatory
High-fiber
Soy-free

Suggested cooking method/program

Grill pan or outdoor grill, stovetop for warming wraps

Storage & meal prep tips

Wraps can be assembled up to 1 day ahead and stored tightly wrapped in parchment or foil in the refrigerator
For best texture, keep slaw and chicken separate and assemble just before eating if prepping more than 1 day ahead

Cortisol reset tip

Turmeric and avocado provide anti-inflammatory compounds and healthy fats to help regulate cortisol and support hormone balance

Possible variations

Add 1/4 cup (35 g) sliced cucumber for extra crunch
Swap cilantro for fresh mint or basil
Use rotisserie chicken for a shortcut
Add 1 tablespoon (10 g) toasted pumpkin seeds for extra magnesium

58. Salmon Niçoise Lettuce Bowl with Lemon-Turmeric Dressing

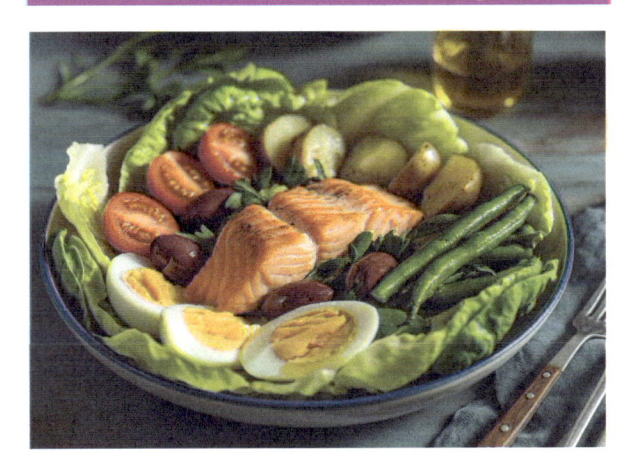

servings: 2

Ingredients

- 2 (4-ounce / 115 g each) wild-caught salmon fillets
- 1 tablespoon (15 ml) extra-virgin olive oil
- 1/2 teaspoon (1 g) ground turmeric
- 1/2 teaspoon (2 g) fine sea salt
- 1/4 teaspoon (0.5 g) ground black pepper
- 4 cups (120 g) mixed baby lettuce leaves
- 1 cup (150 g) cherry tomatoes, halved
- 1/2 cup (70 g) steamed green beans, cut into 2-inch pieces
- 1/2 cup (80 g) cooked baby potatoes, quartered
- 1/4 cup (35 g) pitted Kalamata olives, halved
- 2 large eggs
- 2 tablespoons (8 g) fresh parsley, chopped
- Optional swaps: Use canned wild salmon (drained) for no-cook; swap eggs for chickpeas for vegan; use arugula or spinach for lettuce; omit potatoes for low-carb

Directions

1. Bring a small saucepan of water to a boil. Gently lower eggs into water and boil for 8 minutes for jammy yolks. Transfer to ice water, peel, and halve
2. While eggs cook, pat salmon fillets dry. Rub with olive oil, turmeric, sea salt, and black pepper
3. Heat a nonstick skillet over medium-high. Add salmon, skin-side down, and cook 3–4 minutes per side, until just cooked through and flakes easily. Remove from heat and let rest 2 minutes
4. In a small bowl, whisk together lemon juice, olive oil, Dijon mustard, turmeric, sea salt, and black pepper for the dressing

5. Arrange lettuce in two wide bowls. Top each with cherry tomatoes, green beans, potatoes, olives, and halved eggs
6. Flake salmon into large pieces and arrange on top of each bowl
7. Drizzle with lemon-turmeric dressing and sprinkle with parsley
8. Serve immediately

Lemon-turmeric dressing

2 tablespoons (30 ml) fresh lemon juice
1 tablespoon (15 ml) extra-virgin olive oil
1 teaspoon (5 ml) Dijon mustard
1/2 teaspoon (1 g) ground turmeric
1/4 teaspoon (1 g) fine sea salt
1/4 teaspoon (0.5 g) ground black pepper

Estimated total time

Prep time: 15 minutes
Cook time: 10 minutes
Total: 25 minutes

Nutritional facts per serving

Calories: 410
Protein: 32 g
Fat: 22 g
Carbs: 23 g
Fiber: 6 g
Sugar: 4 g

Dietary labels/tags

Gluten-free
Dairy-free
Anti-inflammatory
High-protein
Soy-free

Suggested cooking method/program

Stovetop skillet for salmon
Stovetop boiling for eggs and potatoes

Storage & meal prep tips

Store components separately in airtight containers in the refrigerator for up to 2 days
Assemble bowls just before serving for best texture
Dressing can be made ahead and refrigerated for up to 5 days

Cortisol reset tip

Wild salmon and eggs provide omega-3s and choline to support brain health and hormone balance, while turmeric and leafy greens help reduce inflammation and support steady energy

Possible variations

Add 1/2 avocado, sliced, for extra healthy fats
Swap green beans for steamed asparagus or snap peas
Use roasted sweet potato cubes instead of baby potatoes
Top with 1 tablespoon (10 g) toasted pumpkin seeds for extra magnesium

59. Mediterranean Eggplant, Quinoa & Walnut Lunch Bowl

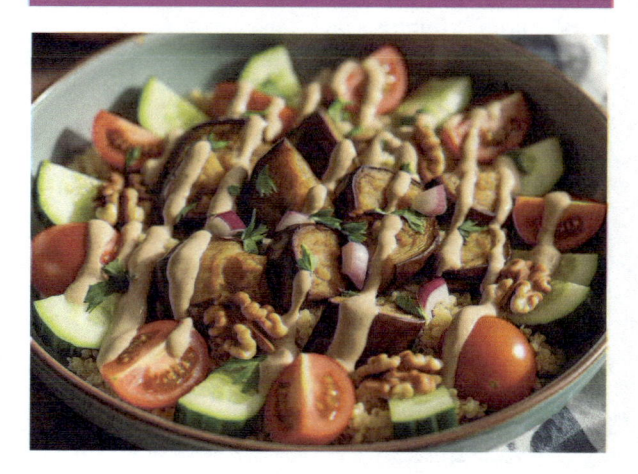

servings: 2

Ingredients

- 1 medium (about 1 lb / 450 g) eggplant, cut into 1-inch cubes
- 2 tablespoons (30 ml) extra-virgin olive oil
- 1/2 teaspoon (2 g) fine sea salt
- 1/4 teaspoon (0.5 g) ground black pepper
- 1/2 teaspoon (1 g) dried oregano
- 1/2 teaspoon (1 g) ground cumin
- 1/2 cup (90 g) dry quinoa, rinsed
- 1 cup (240 ml) low-sodium vegetable broth or water
- 1 cup (150 g) cherry tomatoes, halved
- 1/2 cup (80 g) cucumber, diced
- 1/4 cup (30 g) red onion, finely diced
- 1/4 cup (30 g) raw walnuts, roughly chopped
- 2 tablespoons (8 g) fresh parsley, chopped
- 2 tablespoons (30 ml) fresh lemon juice
- 1 tablespoon (15 ml) tahini
- 1 tablespoon (15 ml) water
- 1 teaspoon (5 ml) pure maple syrup
- Optional swaps: Use brown rice or millet instead of quinoa; swap walnuts for pumpkin seeds for nut-free; omit onion for low-FODMAP; use avocado instead of tahini for a creamy dressing

Directions

1. Preheat oven to 425°F (220°C). Line a baking sheet with parchment paper
2. In a large bowl, toss eggplant cubes with 1 tablespoon olive oil, sea salt, black pepper, oregano, and cumin. Spread evenly on the prepared baking sheet
3. Roast eggplant for 20 minutes, stirring halfway, until golden and tender
4. While eggplant roasts, combine quinoa and vegetable broth in a small saucepan. Bring to a boil, reduce heat to low, cover, and simmer for 15 minutes or until liquid is absorbed. Remove from heat and let stand 5 minutes, then fluff with a fork
5. In a small bowl, whisk together lemon juice, tahini, remaining 1 tablespoon olive oil, water, and maple syrup until smooth
6. In two wide bowls, divide cooked quinoa. Top each with roasted eggplant, cherry tomatoes, cucumber, red onion, and walnuts
7. Drizzle with tahini-lemon dressing and sprinkle with parsley
8. Serve warm or at room temperature

Estimated total time

Prep time: 15 minutes
Cook time: 20 minutes
Total: 35 minutes

Nutritional facts per serving

Calories: 410
Protein: 11 g
Fat: 25 g
Carbs: 41 g
Fiber: 9 g
Sugar: 8 g

Dietary labels/tags

Gluten-free
Dairy-free
Vegan-friendly
Anti-inflammatory
High-fiber

Suggested cooking method/program

Oven roasting for eggplant
Stovetop simmering for quinoa

Storage & meal prep tips

Store assembled bowls in airtight containers in the refrigerator for up to 3 days
Keep dressing separate and add just before serving for best texture
Enjoy cold or gently reheat in the microwave

Cortisol reset tip

Eggplant and walnuts provide antioxidants and healthy fats to help reduce inflammation, while quinoa offers steady energy to support balanced cortisol levels

Possible variations

Add 1/2 cup (80 g) cooked chickpeas for extra protein
Swap parsley for fresh mint or basil
Top with 2 tablespoons (20 g) crumbled feta if dairy is tolerated
Use roasted zucchini or bell pepper in place of eggplant for variety

NOURISHING DINNERS

SHEET PAN AND ONE-POT MEALS

60. Sheet Pan Turmeric Salmon with Roasted Fennel & Sweet Potato

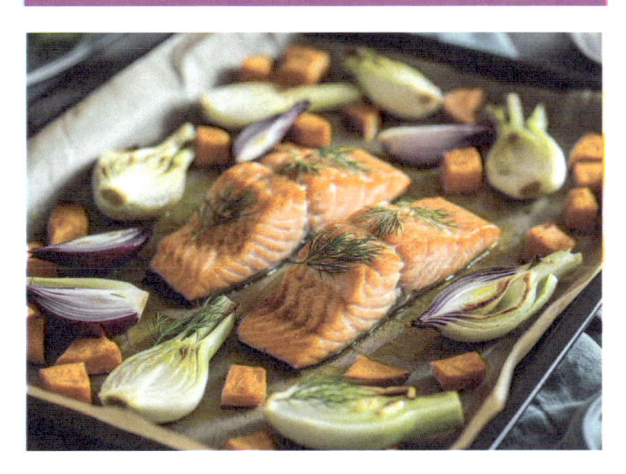

servings: 2

Ingredients

- 2 (4-ounce / 115 g each) wild-caught salmon fillets
- 1 medium (about 8 oz / 225 g) sweet potato, peeled and cut into 1/2-inch cubes
- 1 medium (about 8 oz / 225 g) fennel bulb, trimmed, cored, and sliced into 1/2-inch wedges
- 1 small (about 4 oz / 115 g) red onion, cut into 1/2-inch wedges
- 2 tablespoons (30 ml) extra-virgin olive oil, divided
- 1 teaspoon (2 g) ground turmeric
- 1/2 teaspoon (1 g) smoked paprika
- 1/2 teaspoon (2 g) fine sea salt, divided
- 1/4 teaspoon (0.5 g) ground black pepper
- 1 tablespoon (15 ml) fresh lemon juice
- 2 tablespoons (8 g) fresh dill, chopped
- Optional swaps: Use skinless chicken breast (cut into 1-inch strips) instead of salmon (increase cook time by 5–7 minutes); swap sweet potato for butternut squash; use zucchini or carrots instead of fennel; omit onion for low-FODMAP

Directions

1. Preheat oven to 425°F (220°C). Line a large rimmed sheet pan with parchment paper
2. In a large bowl, toss sweet potato cubes, fennel wedges, and red onion with 1 tablespoon olive oil, 1/4 teaspoon sea salt, and black pepper. Spread evenly on the prepared sheet pan
3. Roast vegetables for 15 minutes
4. While vegetables roast, pat salmon fillets dry. In a small bowl, mix remaining 1 tablespoon olive oil, turmeric, smoked paprika, and 1/4 teaspoon sea salt. Brush mixture over salmon fillets
5. After 15 minutes, remove sheet pan from oven. Push vegetables to the sides and place salmon fillets in the center
6. Return pan to oven and roast for 10 minutes, or until salmon is just cooked through and flakes easily, and vegetables are tender
7. Remove from oven. Drizzle salmon and vegetables with lemon juice and sprinkle with fresh dill
8. Serve immediately

Estimated total time

Prep time: 10 minutes
Cook time: 25 minutes
Total: 35 minutes

Nutritional facts per serving

Calories: 420
Protein: 29 g
Fat: 20 g
Carbs: 34 g
Fiber: 7 g
Sugar: 9 g

Dietary labels/tags

Gluten-free
Dairy-free
Anti-inflammatory
High-protein
Soy-free

Suggested cooking method/program

Sheet pan oven roasting

Storage & meal prep tips

Store cooled salmon and vegetables in separate airtight containers in the refrigerator for up to 2 days
Reheat gently in a 300°F oven or microwave until just warmed through
Best enjoyed fresh for optimal texture

Cortisol reset tip

Turmeric and wild salmon deliver powerful anti-inflammatory benefits, while sweet potato and fennel provide fiber and phytonutrients to support steady energy and hormone balance

Possible variations

Add 1/2 cup (80 g) cooked chickpeas to the pan for extra plant protein

Top with 1 tablespoon (10 g) toasted pumpkin seeds for crunch and magnesium
Swap dill for fresh parsley or basil
Serve over a bed of baby spinach or arugula for extra greens

61. One-Pot Lemon-Ginger Chicken with Quinoa & Kale

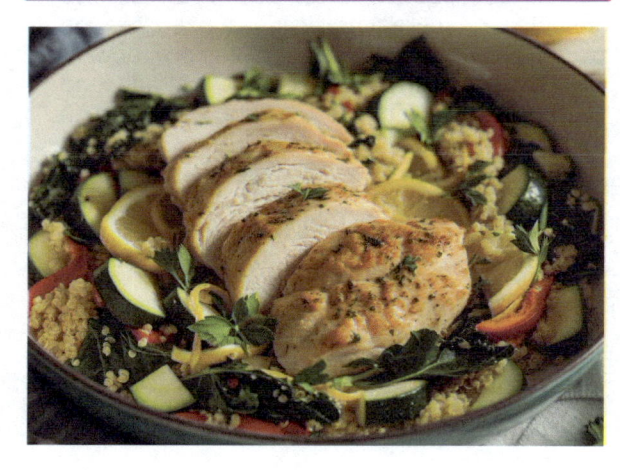

servings: 2

Ingredients

- 2 (5-ounce / 140 g each) boneless, skinless chicken breasts
- 1 tablespoon (15 ml) extra-virgin olive oil
- 1/2 cup (90 g) dry quinoa, rinsed
- 1 1/2 cups (360 ml) low-sodium chicken broth
- 2 cups (60 g) chopped kale, stems removed
- 1 medium (about 4 oz / 115 g) zucchini, diced
- 1/2 cup (75 g) red bell pepper, diced
- 2 cloves garlic, minced
- 1 tablespoon (6 g) fresh ginger, peeled and grated
- 1 teaspoon (2 g) ground turmeric
- 1/2 teaspoon (2 g) fine sea salt
- 1/4 teaspoon (0.5 g) ground black pepper
- Zest and juice of 1 medium lemon (about 2 tablespoons / 30 ml juice)
- 2 tablespoons (8 g) fresh parsley, chopped
- Optional swaps: Use boneless, skinless chicken thighs instead of breasts; swap kale for baby spinach; use vegetable broth for vegetarian (omit chicken, add 1 cup cooked chickpeas); omit garlic for low-FODMAP

Directions

1. Pat chicken breasts dry and season both sides with 1/4 teaspoon salt and black pepper
2. In a large Dutch oven or deep skillet, heat olive oil over medium heat
3. Add chicken breasts and sear 2–3 minutes per side until lightly golden (they will finish cooking later). Remove chicken to a plate
4. Add garlic, ginger, and turmeric to the pot. Sauté 1 minute until fragrant
5. Stir in quinoa, zucchini, and bell pepper. Pour in chicken broth and bring to a gentle boil
6. Nestle chicken breasts back into the pot. Reduce heat to low, cover, and simmer for 15 minutes
7. Remove lid, add kale, lemon zest, and lemon juice. Stir gently, cover, and cook 5–7 minutes more, until quinoa is fluffy, chicken is cooked through (internal temp 165°F), and kale is wilted
8. Remove from heat. Slice chicken and serve bowls topped with parsley

Estimated total time

Prep time: 10 minutes
Cook time: 30 minutes
Total: 40 minutes

Nutritional facts per serving

Calories: 410
Protein: 38 g
Fat: 12 g
Carbs: 38 g
Fiber: 6 g
Sugar: 5 g

Dietary labels/tags

Gluten-free
Dairy-free
Anti-inflammatory
High-protein
One-pot

Suggested cooking method/program

One-pot stovetop simmer

Storage & meal prep tips

Store cooled leftovers in airtight containers in the refrigerator for up to 3 days
Reheat gently on the stovetop with a splash of broth or in the microwave until warmed through
Freeze portions (without kale for best texture) for up to 2 months

Cortisol reset tip

Lemon, ginger, and turmeric offer anti-inflammatory support, while quinoa and kale provide steady energy and micronutrients to help regulate cortisol and support hormone balance

Possible variations

Add 1/2 cup (80 g) cooked chickpeas for extra plant protein
Swap parsley for fresh cilantro or basil
Top with 1 tablespoon (10 g) toasted pumpkin seeds for crunch and magnesium
Use brown rice instead of quinoa (increase simmer time to 35–40 minutes, add more broth as needed)

62. Sheet Pan Harissa Eggplant with Chickpeas & Tahini

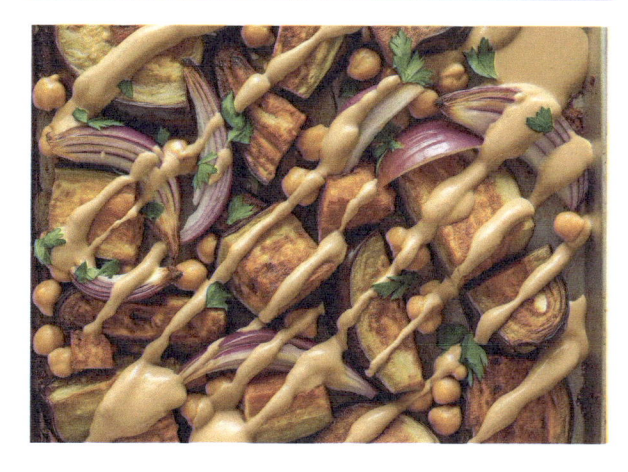

servings: 2

Ingredients

- 1 medium (about 1 lb / 450 g) eggplant, cut into 1-inch cubes
- 1 (15-ounce / 425 g) can no-salt-added chickpeas, drained and rinsed
- 1 small (about 5 oz / 140 g) red onion, cut into 1/2-inch wedges
- 2 tablespoons (30 ml) extra-virgin olive oil
- 1 1/2 tablespoons (24 g) harissa paste (mild or spicy)
- 1/2 teaspoon (2 g) fine sea salt
- 1/4 teaspoon (0.5 g) ground black pepper
- 1/2 teaspoon (1 g) ground cumin
- 1/2 teaspoon (1 g) smoked paprika
- 2 tablespoons (30 ml) tahini
- 1 tablespoon (15 ml) fresh lemon juice
- 2 tablespoons (8 g) fresh parsley, chopped
- Optional swaps: Use zucchini or cauliflower instead of eggplant; swap harissa for mild chili paste or tomato paste with 1/4 teaspoon cayenne; omit onion for low-FODMAP; use sunflower seed butter instead of tahini for nut/seed allergies

Directions

1. Preheat oven to 425°F (220°C). Line a large rimmed sheet pan with parchment paper
2. In a large bowl, toss eggplant cubes, chickpeas, and red onion with olive oil, harissa paste, sea salt, black pepper, cumin, and smoked paprika until evenly coated
3. Spread mixture in a single layer on the prepared sheet pan
4. Roast for 25–30 minutes, stirring halfway, until eggplant is golden and tender and chickpeas are crisp
5. In a small bowl, whisk together tahini and lemon juice with 1 tablespoon (15 ml) water until smooth and pourable
6. Remove sheet pan from oven. Drizzle roasted vegetables and chickpeas with tahini-lemon sauce
7. Sprinkle with fresh parsley and serve warm

Estimated total time

Prep time: 10 minutes
Cook time: 30 minutes
Total: 40 minutes

Nutritional facts per serving

Calories: 390
Protein: 13 g
Fat: 18 g
Carbs: 47 g
Fiber: 13 g
Sugar: 10 g

Dietary labels/tags

Gluten-free
Dairy-free
Vegan
Anti-inflammatory
High-fiber
Soy-free

Suggested cooking method/program

Sheet pan oven roasting

Storage & meal prep tips

Store cooled leftovers in an airtight container in the refrigerator for up to 3 days
Reheat in a 350°F oven or microwave until warmed through
Tahini sauce may thicken in the fridge; thin with a splash of water before serving

Cortisol reset tip

Eggplant and chickpeas provide fiber and plant-based protein to support steady blood sugar, while harissa and tahini offer anti-inflammatory phytonutrients to help regulate stress hormones

Possible variations

Add 1/2 cup (80 g) cherry tomatoes to the pan for extra antioxidants
Top with 1 tablespoon (10 g) toasted pumpkin seeds for crunch and magnesium
Serve over a bed of baby spinach or arugula for extra greens
Swap parsley for fresh cilantro or mint

63. One-Pot Coconut Miso Shrimp with Brown Rice & Baby Bok Choy

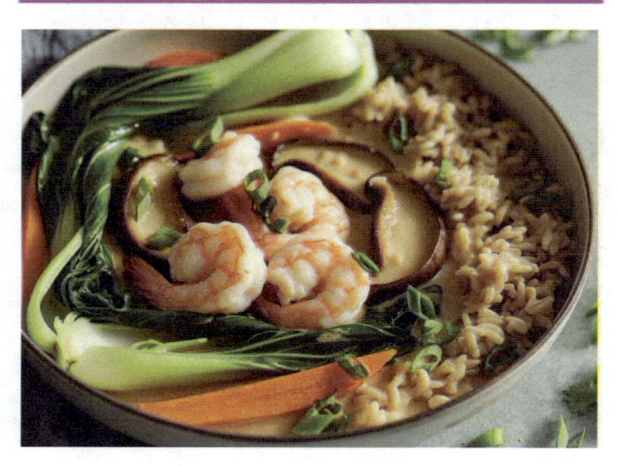

servings: 2

Ingredients

- 1/2 cup (90 g) short-grain brown rice, rinsed
- 1 1/4 cups (300 ml) low-sodium vegetable broth
- 1 (13.5-ounce / 400 ml) can unsweetened light coconut milk
- 2 tablespoons (30 g) white or yellow miso paste
- 1 tablespoon (15 ml) avocado oil or extra-virgin olive oil
- 2 cloves garlic, minced
- 1 tablespoon (6 g) fresh ginger, peeled and grated
- 8 ounces (225 g) raw large shrimp, peeled and deveined
- 2 small (about 6 oz / 170 g total) baby bok choy, halved lengthwise
- 1/2 cup (50 g) shredded carrots
- 1/2 cup (30 g) sliced shiitake mushrooms
- 1/4 teaspoon (2 g) fine sea salt
- 1/4 teaspoon (0.5 g) ground black pepper
- 2 tablespoons (8 g) fresh cilantro or scallions, chopped
- Optional swaps: Use firm tofu cubes (8 oz / 225 g) instead of shrimp for vegan; swap brown rice for white jasmine rice (reduce cook time by 10 minutes); use spinach instead of bok choy; omit garlic for low-FODMAP

Directions

1. In a medium Dutch oven or deep saucepan, combine rinsed brown rice and vegetable broth. Bring to a boil over medium-high heat
2. Reduce heat to low, cover, and simmer for 20 minutes
3. In a small bowl, whisk coconut milk and miso paste until smooth
4. After 20 minutes, uncover pot and stir in coconut-miso mixture, avocado oil, garlic, and ginger
5. Add shrimp, bok choy halves (cut side down), carrots, and mushrooms. Sprinkle with salt and black pepper
6. Cover and simmer on low for 5–7 minutes, until shrimp are opaque and pink, rice is tender, and bok choy is wilted
7. Remove from heat. Gently fluff rice and vegetables with a fork
8. Serve bowls topped with fresh cilantro or scallions

Estimated total time

Prep time: 10 minutes
Cook time: 25 minutes
Total: 35 minutes

Nutritional facts per serving

Calories: 470
Protein: 27 g
Fat: 18 g
Carbs: 52 g
Fiber: 6 g
Sugar: 5 g

Dietary labels/tags

Gluten-free
Dairy-free
Anti-inflammatory
High-protein
One-pot

Suggested cooking method/program

One-pot stovetop simmer

Storage & meal prep tips

Store cooled leftovers in airtight containers in the refrigerator for up to 2 days
Reheat gently on the stovetop with a splash of broth or coconut milk until warmed through

Not recommended for freezing due to shrimp and bok choy texture

Cortisol reset tip

Miso and coconut milk provide gut-friendly probiotics and healthy fats to support hormone balance, while shrimp and brown rice offer steady energy and anti-inflammatory nutrients

Possible variations

Add 1/2 cup (80 g) snap peas or broccoli florets for extra greens
Top with 1 tablespoon (10 g) toasted sesame seeds for crunch and magnesium
Use wild-caught salmon chunks instead of shrimp (simmer 7–8 minutes until cooked through)
Swap cilantro for fresh basil or mint

64. Sheet Pan Herbed Turkey Meatballs with Brussels Sprouts & Cranberry Glaze

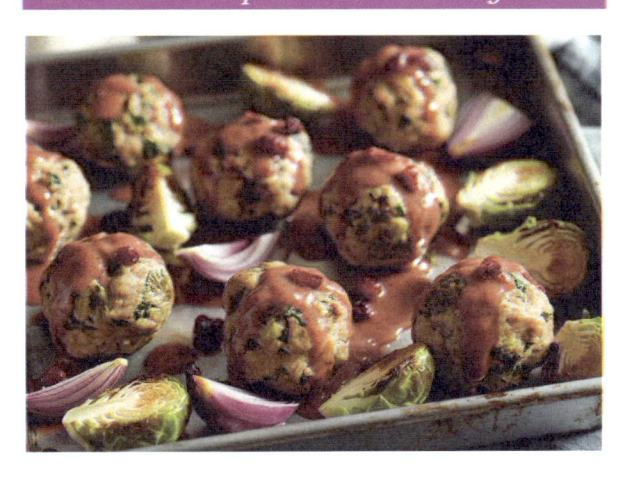

servings: 2

Ingredients

- 8 ounces (225 g) lean ground turkey
- 1/4 cup (20 g) old-fashioned rolled oats
- 1 large egg
- 2 tablespoons (8 g) fresh parsley, finely chopped
- 1 tablespoon (3 g) fresh thyme leaves, chopped
- 1 clove garlic, minced
- 1/2 teaspoon (2 g) fine sea salt
- 1/4 teaspoon (0.5 g) ground black pepper
- 1/2 teaspoon (1 g) dried oregano
- 1 tablespoon (15 ml) extra-virgin olive oil
- 10 ounces (285 g) Brussels sprouts, trimmed and halved
- 1/2 small (60 g) red onion, cut into 1/2-inch wedges
- 1/3 cup (40 g) fresh or frozen cranberries
- 1 tablespoon (15 ml) pure maple syrup
- 1 tablespoon (15 ml) balsamic vinegar
- 1 teaspoon (5 ml) Dijon mustard
- Optional swaps: Use ground chicken instead of turkey; swap oats for gluten-free oats; omit garlic for low-FODMAP; use dried cranberries (unsweetened) if fresh/frozen unavailable

Directions

1. Preheat oven to 425°F (220°C). Line a large rimmed sheet pan with parchment paper
2. In a medium bowl, combine ground turkey, oats, egg, parsley, thyme, garlic, sea salt, black pepper, and oregano. Mix gently with clean hands until just combined
3. Form mixture into 8 equal meatballs (about 1 1/2 tablespoons each) and place on one side of the prepared sheet pan
4. In a separate bowl, toss Brussels sprouts and red onion with olive oil and a pinch of salt and pepper. Spread in a single layer on the other side of the sheet pan
5. Roast for 15 minutes
6. Meanwhile, in a small saucepan over medium heat, combine cranberries, maple syrup, balsamic vinegar, and Dijon mustard. Simmer for 5–7 minutes, stirring occasionally, until cranberries burst and mixture thickens. Mash lightly with a fork
7. After 15 minutes, remove sheet pan from oven. Brush meatballs with half the cranberry glaze
8. Return pan to oven and roast for another 8–10 minutes, until meatballs are cooked through (internal temp 165°F/74°C) and Brussels sprouts are golden
9. Serve meatballs and Brussels sprouts drizzled with remaining cranberry glaze

Estimated total time

Prep time: 15 minutes
Cook time: 25 minutes
Total: 40 minutes

Nutritional facts per serving

Calories: 370
Protein: 28 g
Fat: 15 g
Carbs: 32 g
Fiber: 7 g
Sugar: 10 g

Dietary labels/tags

Gluten-free option
Dairy-free
Anti-inflammatory

High-protein
Sheet pan meal

Suggested cooking method/program

Sheet pan oven roasting

Storage & meal prep tips

Store cooled leftovers in an airtight container in the refrigerator for up to 3 days
Reheat in a 350°F oven or microwave until warmed through
Cranberry glaze may thicken in the fridge; thin with a splash of water if needed

Cortisol reset tip

Turkey provides lean protein to support steady energy and satiety, while Brussels sprouts and cranberries deliver antioxidants and fiber to help reduce inflammation and support hormone balance

Possible variations

Add 1/2 cup (80 g) cubed butternut squash to the pan for extra color and nutrients
Top with 1 tablespoon (10 g) toasted pumpkin seeds for crunch and magnesium
Swap parsley and thyme for fresh sage or rosemary for a different flavor profile
Serve over a bed of baby arugula or quinoa for a more filling meal

LEAN PROTEIN MAINS

65. Lemon-Basil Turkey Cutlets with Sautéed Spinach

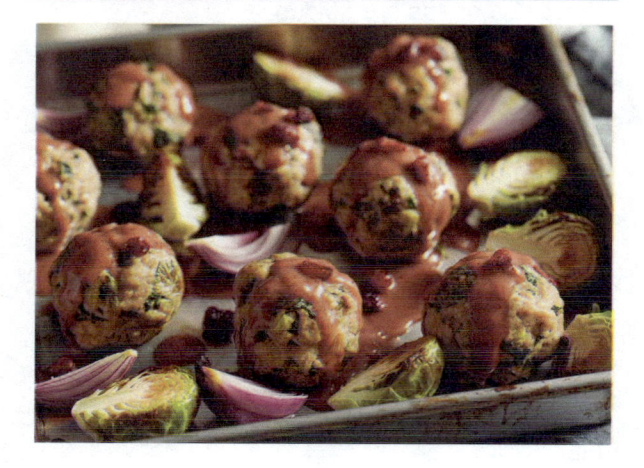

servings: 2

Ingredients

- 8 ounces (225 g) turkey breast cutlets, pounded 1/4-inch thick
- 1/4 teaspoon (2 g) fine sea salt
- 1/4 teaspoon (0.5 g) ground black pepper
- 1 tablespoon (8 g) arrowroot starch or cornstarch
- 1 tablespoon (15 ml) extra-virgin olive oil, divided
- 2 cloves garlic, minced
- 5 ounces (140 g) baby spinach, washed and dried
- 1/4 cup (60 ml) low-sodium chicken broth
- 2 tablespoons (30 ml) freshly squeezed lemon juice
- 1 teaspoon (2 g) lemon zest
- 2 tablespoons (8 g) fresh basil leaves, thinly sliced
- Optional swaps: Use chicken breast cutlets instead of turkey; swap arrowroot for gluten-free flour; omit garlic for low-FODMAP; use baby kale instead of spinach

Directions

1. Pat turkey cutlets dry with paper towels. Season both sides with sea salt and black pepper
2. Place arrowroot starch on a plate. Dredge each cutlet lightly on both sides, shaking off excess
3. Heat 2 teaspoons (10 ml) olive oil in a large nonstick skillet over medium-high heat
4. Add turkey cutlets in a single layer (work in batches if needed). Sear for 2–3 minutes per side, until golden and cooked through (internal temp 165°F/74°C). Transfer to a plate and cover loosely with foil
5. Reduce heat to medium. Add remaining 1 teaspoon (5 ml) olive oil to the skillet
6. Add garlic and sauté for 30 seconds, until fragrant
7. Add baby spinach and toss for 1–2 minutes, until just wilted
8. Pour in chicken broth and lemon juice. Stir, scraping up any browned bits
9. Return turkey cutlets to the skillet. Sprinkle with lemon zest and fresh basil
10. Simmer for 1–2 minutes, spooning sauce over cutlets, until heated through
11. Serve immediately, spooning spinach and pan sauce over turkey

Estimated total time

Prep time: 10 minutes
Cook time: 15 minutes
Total: 25 minutes

Nutritional facts per serving

Calories: 260
Protein: 32 g
Fat: 10 g

Carbs: 8 g
Fiber: 2 g
Sugar: 1 g

Dietary labels/tags

Gluten-free option
Dairy-free
Anti-inflammatory
High-protein
Low-carb

Suggested cooking method/program

Stovetop skillet sauté

Storage & meal prep tips

Store cooled leftovers in an airtight container in the refrigerator for up to 2 days
Reheat gently in a skillet over low heat with a splash of broth or water until warmed through
Not recommended for freezing due to spinach texture

Cortisol reset tip

Lean turkey and spinach provide protein and magnesium to support muscle repair and calm the nervous system, while lemon and basil add antioxidants to help reduce inflammation

Possible variations

Add 1/2 cup (80 g) cherry tomatoes, halved, to the skillet with spinach for extra color and vitamin C
Top with 1 tablespoon (10 g) toasted pine nuts for healthy fats and crunch
Swap basil for fresh parsley or dill for a different herbal note. Serve over a bed of cooked quinoa or cauliflower rice for a more filling meal

66. Miso-Dijon Cod with Wilted Baby Spinach

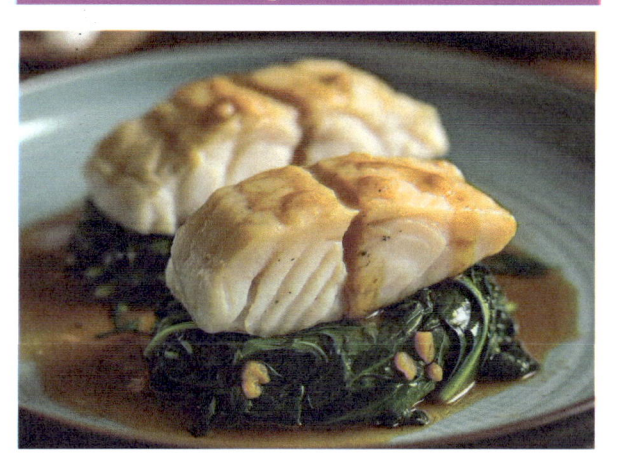

servings: 2

Ingredients

- 2 (5-ounce/140 g each) wild-caught cod fillets, patted dry
- 1 tablespoon (18 g) white miso paste
- 1 tablespoon (15 ml) Dijon mustard
- 1 tablespoon (15 ml) pure maple syrup
- 1 teaspoon (5 ml) rice vinegar
- 1 tablespoon (15 ml) extra-virgin olive oil, divided
- 1/4 teaspoon (2 g) fine sea salt
- 1/4 teaspoon (0.5 g) ground black pepper
- 5 ounces (140 g) baby spinach, washed and dried
- 1 clove garlic, minced
- Optional swaps: Use chickpea miso for soy-free; swap cod for wild Alaskan pollock or haddock; omit garlic for low-FODMAP; use baby kale instead of spinach

Directions

1. Preheat oven to 400°F (200°C). Line a small baking sheet with parchment paper
2. In a small bowl, whisk together miso paste, Dijon mustard, maple syrup, and rice vinegar until smooth
3. Place cod fillets on the prepared baking sheet. Brush each fillet generously with the miso-Dijon glaze, coating the tops and sides
4. Bake cod for 12–14 minutes, until opaque and flakes easily with a fork (internal temp 145°F/63°C)
5. While cod bakes, heat 2 teaspoons (10 ml) olive oil in a large nonstick skillet over medium heat
6. Add minced garlic and sauté for 30 seconds, until fragrant

7. Add baby spinach and a pinch of salt and pepper. Toss for 1–2 minutes, just until wilted
8. Divide wilted spinach between two plates. Top each with a baked cod fillet and drizzle with any remaining pan juices
9. Serve immediately

Estimated total time

Prep time: 10 minutes
Cook time: 15 minutes
Total: 25 minutes

Nutritional facts per serving

Calories: 260
Protein: 28 g
Fat: 9 g
Carbs: 13 g
Fiber: 2 g
Sugar: 6 g

Dietary labels/tags

Gluten-free option
Dairy-free
Anti-inflammatory
High-protein
Low-carb

Suggested cooking method/program

Oven-baked cod, stovetop sautéed spinach

Storage & meal prep tips

Store cooled cod and spinach separately in airtight containers in the refrigerator for up to 2 days
Reheat gently in a 300°F oven or in a covered skillet over low heat until just warmed through
Not recommended for freezing due to spinach texture

Cortisol reset tip

Cod is a lean, easily digestible protein that supports muscle repair and steady energy, while miso and spinach provide antioxidants and minerals to help reduce inflammation and support hormone balance

Possible variations

Top with 1 tablespoon (10 g) toasted sesame seeds for crunch and extra minerals
Add 1/2 cup (80 g) sliced shiitake mushrooms to the skillet with spinach for added fiber and umami
Swap maple syrup for raw honey if preferred
Serve over a bed of cooked quinoa or cauliflower rice for a more filling meal

67. *Ginger-Lime Grilled Mahi-Mahi with Cauliflower Rice*

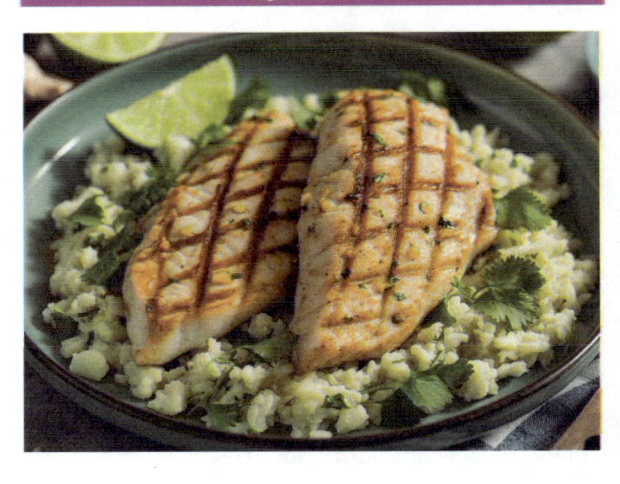

servings: 2

Ingredients

- 2 (5-ounce / 140 g each) wild-caught mahi-mahi fillets, patted dry
- 1 tablespoon (15 ml) avocado oil or extra-virgin olive oil
- 1 tablespoon (15 ml) freshly squeezed lime juice
- 1 teaspoon (2 g) lime zest
- 1 tablespoon (12 g) freshly grated ginger
- 1 clove garlic, minced
- 1/2 teaspoon (3 g) fine sea salt
- 1/4 teaspoon (0.5 g) ground black pepper
- 3 cups (300 g) riced cauliflower (fresh or frozen)
- 1 tablespoon (15 ml) avocado oil or extra-virgin olive oil (for cauliflower rice)
- 2 tablespoons (8 g) fresh cilantro, chopped
- Optional swaps: Use cod or halibut instead of mahi-mahi; omit garlic for low-FODMAP; use parsley instead of cilantro; use coconut oil for a tropical flavor

Directions

1. In a small bowl, whisk together 1 tablespoon oil, lime juice, lime zest, grated ginger, minced garlic, sea salt, and black pepper
2. Place mahi-mahi fillets in a shallow dish or zip-top bag. Pour marinade over fillets, turning to coat. Marinate at room temperature for 10 minutes
3. Preheat a grill or grill pan over medium-high heat. Lightly oil the grates
4. Remove mahi-mahi from marinade, letting excess drip off. Grill fillets for 3–4 minutes per side, until grill marks appear and fish flakes easily with a fork (internal temp 145°F / 63°C)

5. While fish grills, heat 1 tablespoon oil in a large nonstick skillet over medium heat
6. Add riced cauliflower and a pinch of salt. Sauté for 4–5 minutes, stirring occasionally, until tender but not mushy
7. Stir in chopped cilantro and remove from heat
8. Divide cauliflower rice between two plates. Top each with a grilled mahi-mahi fillet
9. Serve immediately, garnished with extra lime wedges if desired

Estimated total time

Prep time: 10 minutes
Cook time: 15 minutes
Total: 25 minutes

Nutritional facts per serving

Calories: 260
Protein: 32 g
Fat: 11 g
Carbs: 8 g
Fiber: 3 g
Sugar: 2 g

Dietary labels/tags

Gluten-free
Dairy-free
Anti-inflammatory
Low-carb
Paleo option

Suggested cooking method/program

Outdoor grill or stovetop grill pan for fish, stovetop sauté for cauliflower rice

Storage & meal prep tips

Store cooled mahi-mahi and cauliflower rice separately in airtight containers in the refrigerator for up to 2 days
Reheat gently in a covered skillet over low heat with a splash of water or broth until just warmed through
Not recommended for freezing due to fish and cauliflower texture

Cortisol reset tip

Mahi-mahi is a lean, high-protein fish rich in B vitamins to support energy and stress resilience, while ginger and lime provide antioxidants to help reduce inflammation

Possible variations

Top with 1 tablespoon (10 g) toasted pumpkin seeds for crunch and extra magnesium
Add 1/2 cup (80 g) diced bell pepper to the cauliflower rice for color and vitamin C
Swap cilantro for fresh basil or mint for a different herbal note
Serve with a side of steamed broccoli or sautéed greens for extra fiber

68. Herb-Crusted Baked Haddock with Roasted Fennel & Lemon

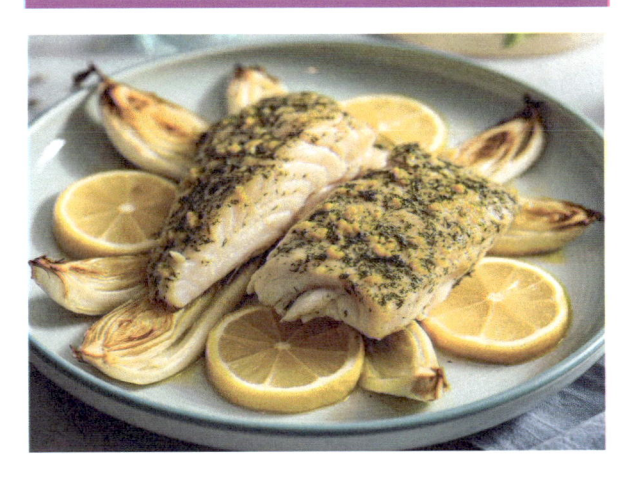

servings: 2

Ingredients

- 2 (5-ounce / 140 g each) wild-caught haddock fillets, patted dry
- 1 tablespoon (15 ml) extra-virgin olive oil, divided
- 1 tablespoon (6 g) finely chopped fresh parsley
- 1 tablespoon (6 g) finely chopped fresh dill
- 1 teaspoon (1 g) finely chopped fresh thyme leaves
- 1 teaspoon (2 g) lemon zest
- 1/2 teaspoon (2 g) fine sea salt, divided
- 1/4 teaspoon (0.5 g) ground black pepper, divided
- 1/2 cup (30 g) almond flour
- 1 large fennel bulb (about 12 ounces / 340 g), trimmed and sliced into 1/2-inch wedges
- 1 small lemon, thinly sliced
- 1 teaspoon (5 ml) fresh lemon juice
- Optional swaps: Use gluten-free panko instead of almond flour; swap haddock for cod or pollock; use dried herbs (1/3 the amount) if fresh are unavailable; omit fennel for low-FODMAP and use zucchini rounds

Directions

1. Preheat oven to 400°F (200°C). Line a large baking sheet with parchment paper

2. Arrange fennel wedges and lemon slices on the baking sheet. Drizzle with 2 teaspoons (10 ml) olive oil and sprinkle with 1/4 teaspoon salt and 1/8 teaspoon pepper. Toss to coat and spread in a single layer
3. Roast fennel and lemon for 10 minutes
4. While vegetables roast, in a shallow bowl, combine almond flour, parsley, dill, thyme, lemon zest, 1/4 teaspoon salt, and 1/8 teaspoon pepper
5. Brush haddock fillets with remaining 1 teaspoon (5 ml) olive oil and a squeeze of lemon juice
6. Press each fillet into the herb-almond mixture, coating both sides well
7. After 10 minutes, remove baking sheet from oven. Push fennel and lemon to the sides and place coated haddock fillets in the center
8. Return to oven and bake for 12 minutes, until fish is opaque and flakes easily with a fork (internal temp 145°F / 63°C) and fennel is golden and tender
9. Serve immediately, dividing roasted fennel and lemon between plates and topping with herb-crusted haddock

Estimated total time

Prep time: 12 minutes
Cook time: 22 minutes
Total: 34 minutes

Nutritional facts per serving

Calories: 295
Protein: 29 g
Fat: 14 g
Carbs: 13 g
Fiber: 4 g
Sugar: 4 g

Dietary labels/tags

Gluten-free
Dairy-free
Anti-inflammatory
Low-carb
Paleo option

Suggested cooking method/program

Oven-roasted, one-pan meal

Storage & meal prep tips

Store cooled haddock and fennel separately in airtight containers in the refrigerator for up to 2 days
Reheat gently in a 300°F oven or covered skillet over low heat until just warmed through
Not recommended for freezing due to texture changes

Cortisol reset tip

Haddock is a lean, easily digestible protein that supports muscle repair and steady energy, while fennel and fresh herbs provide antioxidants and phytonutrients to help reduce inflammation and support hormone balance

Possible variations

Top with 1 tablespoon (10 g) toasted pine nuts for extra crunch and healthy fats
Add 1/2 cup (80 g) cherry tomatoes to the baking sheet for color and vitamin C
Swap almond flour for ground sunflower seeds for a nut-free version
Serve over a bed of baby arugula or spinach for extra greens

69. Cedar-Plank Lemon Trout with Steamed Asparagus

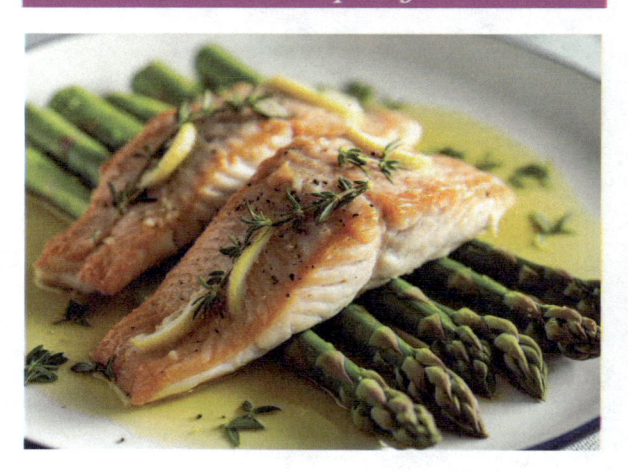

servings: 2

Ingredients

- 2 (5-ounce / 140 g each) boneless skin-on trout fillets, patted dry
- 1 untreated cedar plank (about 12 x 6 inches), soaked in water for at least 1 hour
- 1 tablespoon (15 ml) extra-virgin olive oil
- 1 tablespoon (15 ml) freshly squeezed lemon juice
- 1 teaspoon (2 g) lemon zest
- 1 teaspoon (2 g) fresh thyme leaves, chopped
- 1/2 teaspoon (3 g) fine sea salt, divided
- 1/4 teaspoon (0.5 g) ground black pepper, divided
- 1 bunch (about 12 ounces / 340 g) fresh asparagus, trimmed

- 1 teaspoon (5 ml) extra-virgin olive oil (for asparagus)
- 1 tablespoon (4 g) fresh parsley, chopped
- Optional swaps: Use salmon fillets instead of trout; swap thyme for dill or tarragon; use ghee instead of olive oil; omit lemon zest for low-FODMAP

Directions

1. Preheat an outdoor grill to medium (about 400°F) or preheat oven to 400°F (200°C).
2. In a small bowl, combine 1 tablespoon olive oil, lemon juice, lemon zest, thyme, 1/4 teaspoon salt, and 1/8 teaspoon pepper.
3. Place trout fillets skin-side down on a plate. Brush tops evenly with lemon-herb mixture.
4. Place soaked cedar plank on grill grates or in oven for 2 minutes, then carefully remove and arrange trout fillets skin-side down on the plank.
5. Return plank with trout to grill or oven. Close lid (or oven door) and cook for 12–15 minutes, until trout is opaque and flakes easily with a fork (internal temp 145°F / 63°C).
6. While trout cooks, fill a large skillet with 1 inch of water and bring to a simmer over medium-high heat.
7. Add asparagus in a single layer, cover, and steam for 3–4 minutes until bright green and just tender. Drain and toss with 1 teaspoon olive oil, 1/4 teaspoon salt, and 1/8 teaspoon pepper.
8. Transfer steamed asparagus to plates. Top with chopped parsley.
9. Carefully remove trout from cedar plank and serve alongside asparagus.

Estimated total time

Prep time: 15 minutes
Cook time: 20 minutes
Total: 35 minutes

Nutritional facts per serving

Calories: 265
Protein: 29 g
Fat: 13 g
Carbs: 8 g
Fiber: 3 g
Sugar: 3 g

Dietary labels/tags

Gluten-free
Dairy-free
Anti-inflammatory
Low-carb
Paleo option

Suggested cooking method/program

Cedar plank grilling or oven-roasting for trout, stovetop steaming for asparagus

Storage & meal prep tips

Store cooled trout and asparagus separately in airtight containers in the refrigerator for up to 2 days
Reheat trout gently in a 300°F oven or covered skillet over low heat until just warmed through
Not recommended for freezing due to texture changes

Cortisol reset tip

Trout is rich in omega-3s and vitamin D, both of which help regulate inflammation and support mood balance, while asparagus provides prebiotic fiber for gut health and hormone support

Possible variations

Top trout with 1 tablespoon (10 g) toasted sliced almonds for extra crunch and magnesium
Add 1/2 cup (80 g) cherry tomatoes to the asparagus for color and vitamin C
Swap parsley for fresh basil or chives for a different herbal note
Serve with a side of quinoa or wild rice for extra fiber and minerals

PLANT-BASED GENTLE OPTIONS

70. Miso-Maple Roasted Carrot & Lentil Bowl

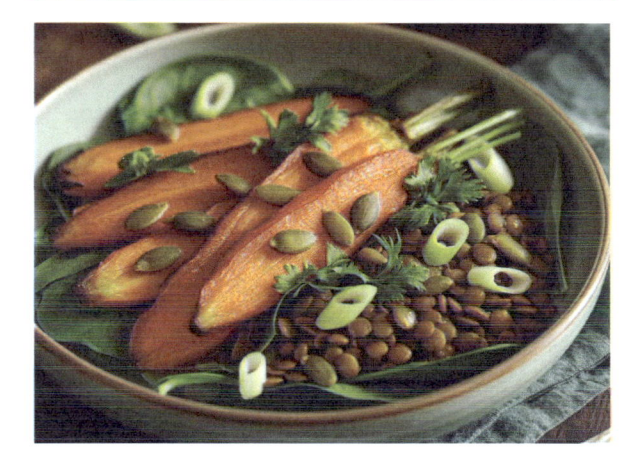

servings: 2

Ingredients

- 1 pound (450 g) medium carrots, peeled and cut into 1/2-inch diagonal slices
- 1 tablespoon (15 ml) extra-virgin olive oil

- 1 tablespoon (18 g) white or yellow miso paste
- 1 tablespoon (15 ml) pure maple syrup
- 1 tablespoon (15 ml) apple cider vinegar
- 1/2 teaspoon (2 g) fine sea salt, divided
- 1/4 teaspoon (0.5 g) ground black pepper, divided
- 1 cup (200 g) cooked green or brown lentils (from 1/2 cup dry)
- 2 cups (60 g) baby spinach, packed
- 1/4 cup (30 g) raw pumpkin seeds (pepitas)
- 1/4 cup (25 g) thinly sliced scallions (green onions)
- 1 tablespoon (4 g) chopped fresh cilantro or parsley
- Optional swaps: Use gluten-free chickpea miso for soy-free; swap maple syrup for raw honey; use arugula or baby kale instead of spinach; omit pumpkin seeds for nut-free

Directions

1. Preheat oven to 425°F (220°C). Line a large rimmed baking sheet with parchment paper
2. In a large bowl, whisk together olive oil, miso paste, maple syrup, apple cider vinegar, 1/4 teaspoon salt, and 1/8 teaspoon pepper until smooth
3. Add carrot slices to the bowl and toss to coat evenly
4. Spread carrots in a single layer on the prepared baking sheet
5. Roast for 25–30 minutes, stirring halfway, until carrots are caramelized and tender
6. While carrots roast, rinse and drain cooked lentils if using canned; warm gently in a small saucepan with 2 tablespoons (30 ml) water and 1/4 teaspoon salt over low heat for 3–4 minutes
7. Divide baby spinach between two wide bowls
8. Top each bowl with warm lentils, roasted carrots, pumpkin seeds, scallions, and chopped herbs
9. Sprinkle with remaining black pepper and serve immediately

Estimated total time

Prep time: 15 minutes
Cook time: 30 minutes
Total: 45 minutes

Nutritional facts per serving

Calories: 340
Protein: 13 g
Fat: 12 g
Carbs: 48 g
Fiber: 12 g
Sugar: 13 g

Dietary labels/tags

Gluten-free
Dairy-free
Vegan
Anti-inflammatory
High-fiber

Suggested cooking method/program

Oven-roasted, one-pan meal

Storage & meal prep tips

Store cooled components separately in airtight containers in the refrigerator for up to 3 days
Reheat carrots and lentils gently in a skillet over low heat or in the microwave before assembling bowls
Not recommended for freezing due to texture changes

Cortisol reset tip

Carrots and lentils provide steady, plant-based energy and prebiotic fiber to support gut health and hormone balance, while miso offers fermented probiotics for a calmer, more resilient stress response

Possible variations

Top with 1/4 avocado per bowl for extra healthy fats
Add 1/2 cup (80 g) roasted beets or sweet potato for more color and antioxidants
Swap pumpkin seeds for sunflower seeds or hemp hearts. Drizzle with 1 teaspoon tahini or plain coconut yogurt for a creamy finish

71. Silken Tofu & Wakame Miso Broth with Greens

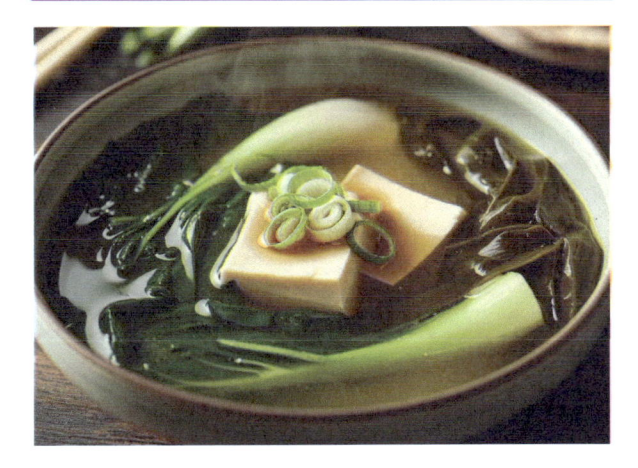

servings: 2

Ingredients

- 3 cups (720 ml) filtered water
- 2 tablespoons (18 g) white or yellow miso paste
- 1/2 ounce (14 g) dried wakame seaweed
- 6 ounces (170 g) silken tofu, drained and cut into 1/2-inch cubes
- 2 cups (60 g) baby bok choy, chopped
- 1 cup (30 g) baby spinach, packed
- 2 scallions (20 g), thinly sliced
- 1 teaspoon (5 ml) toasted sesame oil
- 1/4 teaspoon (1 g) fine sea salt, or to taste
- 1/8 teaspoon (0.25 g) ground white pepper
- Optional swaps: Use chickpea miso for soy-free; swap bok choy for napa cabbage or Swiss chard; omit sesame oil for oil-free; use firm tofu for more texture

Directions

1. In a medium saucepan, bring 3 cups filtered water to a gentle simmer over medium heat
2. Add dried wakame and simmer for 3 minutes until rehydrated and tender
3. Reduce heat to low. In a small bowl, whisk miso paste with 1/4 cup (60 ml) hot broth from the pot until smooth, then stir back into the saucepan
4. Gently add silken tofu cubes and chopped bok choy. Simmer for 2–3 minutes until bok choy is just wilted
5. Stir in baby spinach and half the sliced scallions. Cook for 1 minute until spinach is bright green
6. Remove from heat. Drizzle with toasted sesame oil, season with sea salt and white pepper
7. Ladle into bowls and garnish with remaining scallions

Estimated total time

Prep time: 10 minutes
Cook time: 10 minutes
Total: 20 minutes

Nutritional facts per serving

Calories: 110
Protein: 8 g
Fat: 5 g
Carbs: 10 g
Fiber: 3 g
Sugar: 2 g

Dietary labels/tags

Gluten-free
Dairy-free
Vegan
Anti-inflammatory
Low-calorie

Suggested cooking method/program

Stovetop, one-pot

Storage & meal prep tips

Store cooled broth in an airtight container in the refrigerator for up to 2 days
Reheat gently over low heat; avoid boiling to preserve tofu texture
Not recommended for freezing due to tofu and greens texture changes

Cortisol reset tip

Seaweed and miso provide trace minerals and fermented probiotics to support thyroid and adrenal health, while tofu and greens offer plant-based protein and magnesium for steady energy and calm

Possible variations

Add 1/2 cup (75 g) sliced shiitake mushrooms for extra umami and immune support
Top with 1 tablespoon (8 g) hemp seeds for more healthy fats
Swap spinach for watercress or arugula for a peppery twist. Stir in 1/2 teaspoon grated fresh ginger for added anti-inflammatory benefits

72. Avocado-Cucumber Zucchini Noodles with Lemon-Hemp Pesto

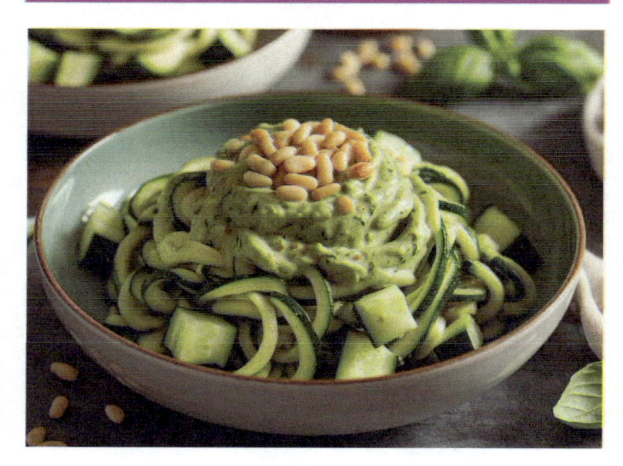

servings: 2

Ingredients

- 2 medium zucchini (about 12 oz/340 g), spiralized into noodles
- 1 ripe avocado (about 6 oz/170 g), peeled and pitted
- 1 cup (130 g) diced English cucumber
- 1 cup (30 g) fresh basil leaves, packed
- 1/4 cup (30 g) raw shelled hemp seeds
- 2 tablespoons (30 ml) fresh lemon juice
- 1 tablespoon (15 ml) extra-virgin olive oil
- 1 small garlic clove (3 g), minced
- 1/2 teaspoon (2 g) fine sea salt, divided
- 1/4 teaspoon (0.5 g) ground black pepper
- 1/4 cup (30 g) toasted pine nuts or pumpkin seeds, for topping
- Optional swaps: Use yellow squash instead of zucchini; swap basil for baby spinach or arugula; omit garlic for low-FODMAP; use sunflower seeds for nut-free

Directions

1. Spiralize zucchini into noodles using a spiralizer or julienne peeler; set aside on a clean kitchen towel to absorb excess moisture
2. In a food processor, combine avocado, basil, hemp seeds, lemon juice, olive oil, garlic, 1/4 teaspoon salt, and black pepper
3. Blend until smooth and creamy, scraping down sides as needed
4. Taste and adjust seasoning with additional salt or lemon juice if desired
5. In a large mixing bowl, gently toss zucchini noodles and cucumber with the avocado-hemp pesto until evenly coated
6. Divide between two wide bowls
7. Sprinkle each serving with toasted pine nuts or pumpkin seeds
8. Serve immediately for best texture

Estimated total time

Prep time: 20 minutes
Cook time: 0 minutes
Total: 20 minutes

Nutritional facts per serving

Calories: 340
Protein: 10 g
Fat: 27 g
Carbs: 19 g
Fiber: 8 g
Sugar: 6 g

Dietary labels/tags

Gluten-free
Dairy-free
Vegan
Anti-inflammatory
Raw
Low-carb

Suggested cooking method/program

No-cook, raw preparation

Storage & meal prep tips

Store pesto and spiralized zucchini separately in airtight containers in the refrigerator for up to 2 days
Toss just before serving to prevent sogginess
Not recommended for freezing due to avocado and zucchini texture changes

Cortisol reset tip

Avocado and hemp seeds provide magnesium and healthy fats to support adrenal health and steady energy, while raw zucchini and cucumber offer hydrating, anti-inflammatory phytonutrients for gentle digestion

Possible variations

Add 1/2 cup (75 g) halved cherry tomatoes for color and vitamin C
Top with 1 tablespoon (8 g) hemp hearts or chia seeds for extra omega-3s
Mix in 1/4 cup (30 g) shredded carrots or radishes for crunch
Swap lemon juice for lime and add cilantro for a fresh twist

SNACKS, SIDES, AND LONG-TERM SUCCESS

ANTI-INFLAMMATORY SNACK RECIPES

73. Turmeric-Spiced Roasted Chickpeas

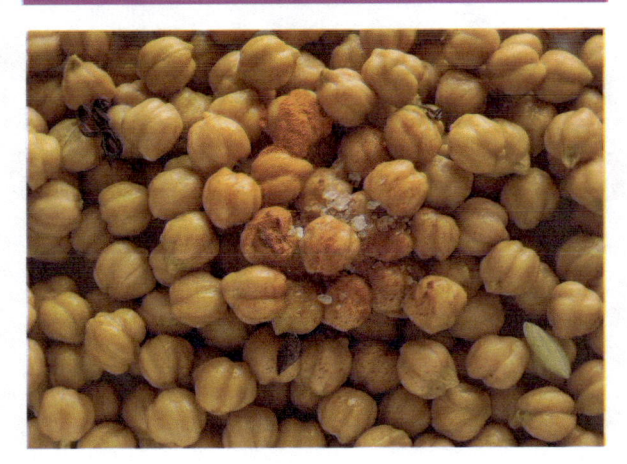

servings: 4

Ingredients

- 1 can (15 oz/425 g) no-salt-added chickpeas, drained and rinsed
- 1 tablespoon (15 ml) extra-virgin olive oil
- 1 teaspoon (2 g) ground turmeric
- 1/2 teaspoon (1 g) ground cumin
- 1/2 teaspoon (1 g) smoked paprika
- 1/4 teaspoon (0.5 g) ground black pepper
- 1/2 teaspoon (2 g) fine sea salt
- 1/4 teaspoon (0.5 g) garlic powder
- Optional swaps: Use avocado oil for a higher smoke point; swap smoked paprika for sweet paprika; omit garlic powder for low-FODMAP; use cooked, cooled chickpeas from scratch for sodium control

Directions

1. Preheat oven to 400°F (205°C). Line a rimmed baking sheet with parchment paper
2. Pat chickpeas very dry with a clean kitchen towel or paper towels to ensure crispiness
3. In a medium bowl, toss chickpeas with olive oil until evenly coated
4. Sprinkle turmeric, cumin, smoked paprika, black pepper, sea salt, and garlic powder over chickpeas
5. Toss again to coat thoroughly with spices
6. Spread chickpeas in a single layer on the prepared baking sheet
7. Roast for 25–30 minutes, shaking the pan halfway through, until golden and crisp
8. Let cool for 10 minutes on the pan before serving for maximum crunch

Estimated total time

Prep time: 10 minutes
Cook time: 30 minutes
Total: 40 minutes

Nutritional facts per serving

Calories: 120
Protein: 5 g
Fat: 5 g
Carbs: 15 g
Fiber: 4 g
Sugar: 1 g

Dietary labels/tags

Gluten-free
Dairy-free
Vegan
Anti-inflammatory
High-fiber

Suggested cooking method/program

Oven-roasted, single sheet pan

Storage & meal prep tips

Store cooled chickpeas in an airtight container at room temperature for up to 2 days
For best texture, do not refrigerate; re-crisp in a 350°F (175°C) oven for 5 minutes if needed

Cortisol reset tip

Turmeric and cumin provide anti-inflammatory phytonutrients that help modulate stress hormones, while chickpeas offer plant-based protein and fiber for steady energy and satiety

Possible variations

Add 1/4 teaspoon (0.5 g) cayenne pepper for a spicy kick
Toss with 1 tablespoon (8 g) sesame seeds before roasting for extra crunch
Use a blend of chickpeas and shelled edamame for more protein. Sprinkle with fresh chopped parsley or cilantro after roasting for a burst of color and antioxidants

74. Lemon-Hemp Seed Kale Chips

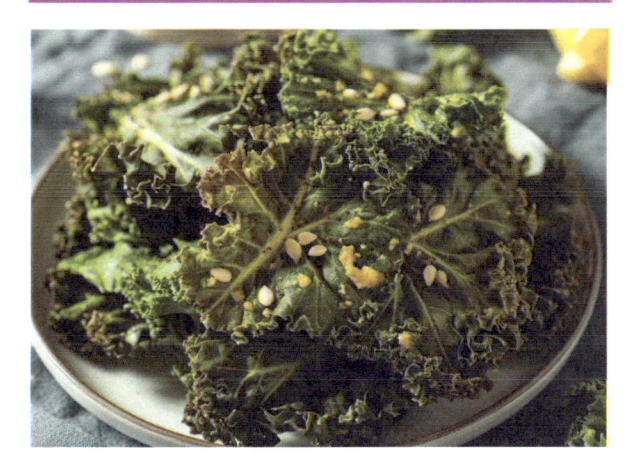

servings: 4

Ingredients

- 1 large bunch curly kale (about 8 oz/225 g), stems removed, leaves torn into 2-inch pieces
- 2 tablespoons (30 ml) extra-virgin olive oil
- 2 tablespoons (20 g) raw shelled hemp seeds
- 1 tablespoon (15 ml) fresh lemon juice
- 1 teaspoon (2 g) lemon zest
- 1/2 teaspoon (2 g) fine sea salt
- 1/4 teaspoon (0.5 g) ground black pepper
- Optional swaps: Use avocado oil for a higher smoke point; swap hemp seeds for ground flaxseed or chia seeds; omit lemon zest for low-FODMAP; use lacinato kale for a milder flavor

Directions

1. Preheat oven to 300°F (150°C). Line a large baking sheet with parchment paper
2. Wash and thoroughly dry kale leaves using a salad spinner or clean kitchen towels
3. In a large bowl, whisk together olive oil, lemon juice, lemon zest, sea salt, and black pepper
4. Add kale pieces to the bowl and massage dressing into leaves for 1–2 minutes until evenly coated and slightly softened
5. Sprinkle hemp seeds over kale and toss gently to distribute
6. Arrange kale in a single layer on the prepared baking sheet, making sure leaves do not overlap
7. Bake for 22–25 minutes, rotating the pan halfway through, until chips are crisp and edges are lightly browned
8. Let cool on the pan for 5 minutes before serving for maximum crunch

Estimated total time

Prep time: 10 minutes
Cook time: 25 minutes
Total: 35 minutes

Nutritional facts per serving

Calories: 110
Protein: 3 g
Fat: 8 g
Carbs: 7 g
Fiber: 2 g
Sugar: 1 g

Dietary labels/tags

Gluten-free
Dairy-free
Vegan
Anti-inflammatory
Nut-free

Suggested cooking method/program

Oven-baked, single sheet pan

Storage & meal prep tips

Store completely cooled chips in an airtight container at room temperature for up to 2 days
If chips lose crispness, re-crisp in a 250°F (120°C) oven for 5 minutes

Cortisol reset tip

Kale and hemp seeds deliver magnesium, vitamin C, and plant-based omega-3s to help regulate stress response and support adrenal health

Possible variations

Add 1/4 teaspoon (0.5 g) smoked paprika or turmeric for extra anti-inflammatory flavor
Sprinkle with 1 tablespoon (8 g) nutritional yeast before baking for a cheesy, B-vitamin boost
Mix in 1/2 teaspoon (2 g) garlic powder for a savory twist. Use baby kale for a more delicate chip

75. Cortisol-Calm Apple Walnut Snack Packs

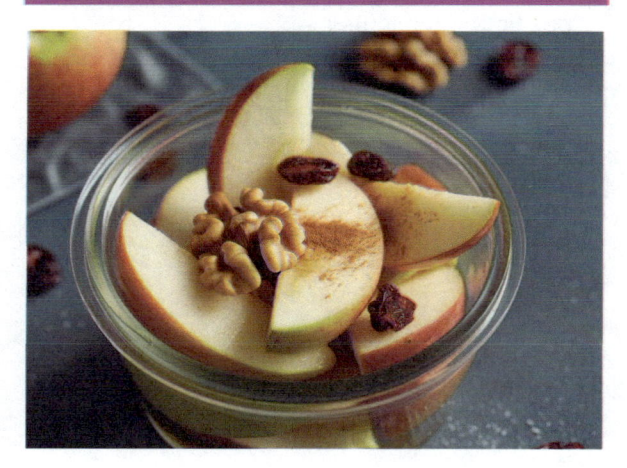

🍽servings: 4

Ingredients

- 2 medium crisp apples (about 7 oz/200 g each), cored and sliced into 1/2-inch wedges
- 1/2 cup (60 g) raw walnut halves
- 2 tablespoons (20 g) unsweetened dried cranberries
- 1 tablespoon (15 ml) fresh lemon juice
- 1/4 teaspoon (1 g) ground cinnamon
- Optional swaps: Use pecans or almonds instead of walnuts; swap dried cranberries for unsweetened dried cherries or blueberries; use sunflower seeds for nut-free; omit cinnamon for low-FODMAP

Directions

1. Place apple slices in a large bowl and toss with lemon juice to prevent browning
2. Sprinkle ground cinnamon evenly over apple slices and toss gently to coat
3. Divide apple slices evenly among 4 small airtight containers or snack bags
4. Add 2 tablespoons (15 g) walnut halves and 1/2 tablespoon (5 g) dried cranberries to each container
5. Seal containers and refrigerate until ready to eat, up to 2 days

Estimated total time

Prep time: 10 minutes
No cook time
Total: 10 minutes

Nutritional facts per serving

Calories: 140
Protein: 2 g
Fat: 10 g
Carbs: 13 g
Fiber: 3 g
Sugar: 8 g

Dietary labels/tags

Gluten-free
Dairy-free
Vegan
Anti-inflammatory
No added sugar

Suggested cooking method/program

No-cook, meal prep/snack pack

Storage & meal prep tips

Store snack packs in airtight containers in the refrigerator for up to 2 days
For best texture, add walnuts just before eating if prepping more than 24 hours ahead

Cortisol reset tip

Walnuts provide plant-based omega-3s and magnesium to help regulate stress response, while apples offer fiber and polyphenols for steady energy and gut health

Possible variations

Add 1 tablespoon (8 g) pumpkin seeds per pack for extra crunch and zinc
Swap apples for firm pear slices for a seasonal twist
Sprinkle with 1 teaspoon (4 g) cacao nibs for a chocolatey antioxidant boost. Use a dash of ground ginger or cardamom instead of cinnamon for a different anti-inflammatory flavor

76. Ginger-Sesame Steamed Edamame

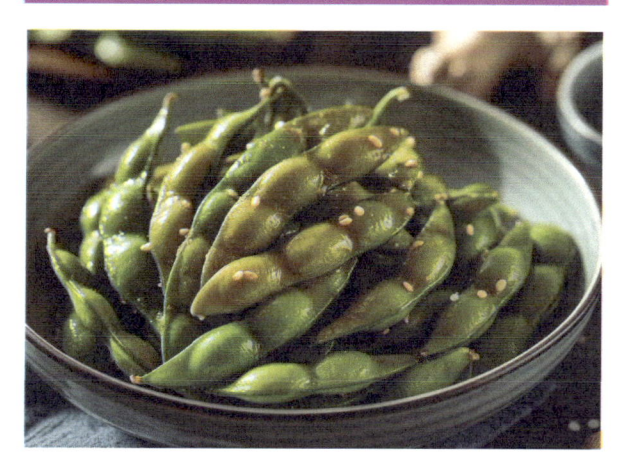

servings: 4

Ingredients

- 2 cups (280 g) frozen edamame in pods
- 1 tablespoon (15 ml) toasted sesame oil
- 1 tablespoon (15 ml) low-sodium tamari or coconut aminos
- 1 teaspoon (5 g) freshly grated ginger
- 1/2 teaspoon (2 g) garlic powder
- 1/2 teaspoon (2 g) fine sea salt
- 1 tablespoon (9 g) toasted sesame seeds
- Optional swaps: Use olive oil instead of sesame oil for sesame allergy; swap tamari for gluten-free soy sauce; omit garlic powder for low-FODMAP; use shelled edamame for easier eating

Directions

1. Add 2 cups (280 g) frozen edamame pods to a steamer basket set over 1 inch of boiling water in a medium saucepan
2. Cover and steam for 6–8 minutes until edamame are bright green and tender
3. While edamame steams, whisk together 1 tablespoon (15 ml) toasted sesame oil, 1 tablespoon (15 ml) tamari, 1 teaspoon (5 g) grated ginger, and 1/2 teaspoon (2 g) garlic powder in a small bowl
4. Transfer steamed edamame to a large bowl
5. Drizzle with sesame-ginger sauce and toss to coat evenly
6. Sprinkle with 1/2 teaspoon (2 g) sea salt and 1 tablespoon (9 g) toasted sesame seeds
7. Serve warm, squeezing pods to pop out beans as you eat

Estimated total time

Prep time: 5 minutes
Cook time: 8 minutes
Total: 13 minutes

Nutritional facts per serving

Calories: 120
Protein: 9 g
Fat: 6 g
Carbs: 10 g
Fiber: 4 g
Sugar: 1 g

Dietary labels/tags

Gluten-free
Dairy-free
Vegan
Anti-inflammatory
High-fiber

Suggested cooking method/program

Steamed, stovetop

Storage & meal prep tips

Store cooled edamame in an airtight container in the refrigerator for up to 3 days
Reheat gently in the microwave or enjoy cold as a snack or salad topper

Cortisol reset tip

Edamame provides plant-based protein and magnesium to help stabilize blood sugar and support adrenal function, while ginger and sesame oil offer anti-inflammatory benefits

Possible variations

Add 1/2 teaspoon (2 g) chili flakes for a spicy kick
Toss with 1 tablespoon (8 g) chopped fresh cilantro for extra freshness
Use shelled edamame and serve over brown rice for a quick lunch. Sprinkle with 1 teaspoon (4 g) lemon zest for a citrusy twist

77. No-Bake Almond-Cacao Energy Squares

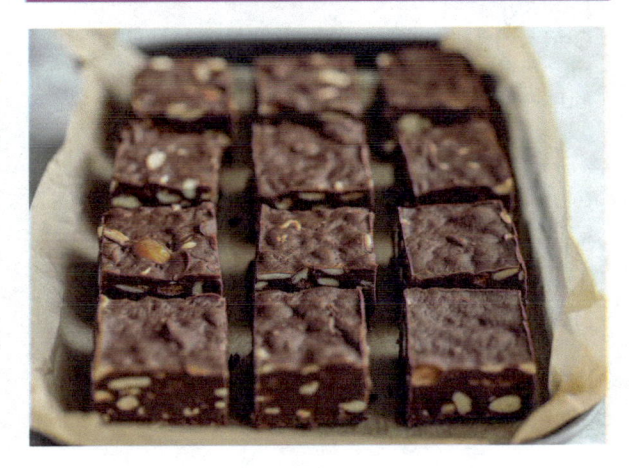

servings: 12 squares

Ingredients

- 1 cup (140 g) raw almonds
- 1/2 cup (45 g) rolled oats (use certified gluten-free if needed)
- 1/4 cup (20 g) unsweetened cacao powder
- 1/2 cup (80 g) Medjool dates, pitted (about 5–6 large dates)
- 2 tablespoons (30 ml) pure maple syrup
- 1 tablespoon (15 ml) coconut oil, melted
- 1/4 teaspoon (1 g) fine sea salt
- 1 teaspoon (5 ml) pure vanilla extract
- Optional swaps: Use walnuts or cashews instead of almonds; swap maple syrup for raw honey; use sunflower seeds for nut-free; omit oats for grain-free; use carob powder for caffeine-free

Directions

1. Line an 8x4-inch loaf pan with parchment paper, leaving overhang for easy removal
2. Add almonds and oats to a food processor; pulse 8–10 times until coarsely chopped
3. Add cacao powder, pitted dates, maple syrup, coconut oil, sea salt, and vanilla extract
4. Process for 1–2 minutes, scraping down sides as needed, until mixture is sticky and holds together when pressed
5. Transfer mixture to prepared pan; press firmly and evenly into all corners using a spatula or damp hands
6. Chill in the refrigerator for at least 1 hour to set
7. Lift out using parchment overhang; cut into 12 squares
8. Store in an airtight container in the refrigerator for up to 1 week

Estimated total time

Prep time: 12 minutes
No cook time
Total: 12 minutes

Nutritional facts per serving

Calories: 120
Protein: 3 g
Fat: 7 g
Carbs: 13 g
Fiber: 3 g
Sugar: 7 g

Dietary labels/tags

Gluten-free (if using GF oats)
Dairy-free
Vegan
Anti-inflammatory
No added refined sugar

Suggested cooking method/program

No-bake, food processor

Storage & meal prep tips

Store squares in an airtight container in the refrigerator for up to 1 week
For longer storage, freeze for up to 2 months and thaw as needed

Cortisol reset tip

Almonds and cacao provide magnesium and polyphenols to help regulate stress hormones and support mood, while dates offer natural sweetness and fiber for steady energy

Possible variations

Add 2 tablespoons (16 g) chia seeds or hemp hearts for extra omega-3s
Mix in 1/4 cup (40 g) mini dark chocolate chips for a treat
Swap almonds for pumpkin seeds for a nut-free version
Sprinkle with flaky sea salt before chilling for a sweet-salty finish

SMART BEVERAGES & HEALING INFUSION RECIPES

78. Sleep-Reset Turmeric Golden Milk

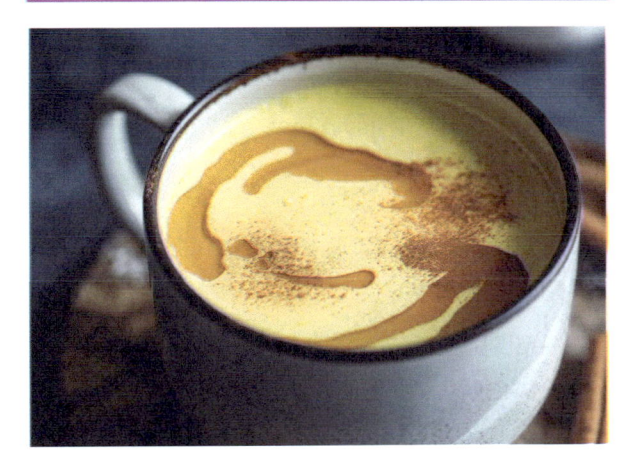

servings: 2

Ingredients

- 2 cups (480 ml) unsweetened almond milk (or other non-dairy milk)
- 1 tablespoon (15 ml) pure maple syrup
- 1 teaspoon (2 g) ground turmeric
- 1/2 teaspoon (1 g) ground cinnamon
- 1/4 teaspoon (0.5 g) ground ginger
- 1/8 teaspoon (0.5 g) ground black pepper
- 1 teaspoon (5 ml) coconut oil
- 1/2 teaspoon (2 ml) pure vanilla extract
- Optional swaps: Use oat or cashew milk for creamier texture; swap maple syrup for raw honey; omit black pepper for low-FODMAP; use fresh grated turmeric and ginger (1 teaspoon each) for extra potency

Directions

1. Add 2 cups (480 ml) almond milk to a small saucepan
2. Whisk in 1 tablespoon (15 ml) maple syrup, 1 teaspoon (2 g) turmeric, 1/2 teaspoon (1 g) cinnamon, 1/4 teaspoon (1 g) ginger, and 1/8 teaspoon (0.5 g) black pepper
3. Stir in 1 teaspoon (5 ml) coconut oil
4. Heat over medium-low, whisking frequently, until steaming hot but not boiling (about 4–5 minutes)
5. Remove from heat and stir in 1/2 teaspoon (2 ml) vanilla extract
6. Pour into mugs and serve warm

Estimated total time

Prep time: 5 minutes
Cook time: 5 minutes
Total: 10 minutes

Nutritional facts per serving

Calories: 90
Protein: 1 g
Fat: 5 g
Carbs: 11 g
Fiber: 1 g
Sugar: 7 g

Dietary labels/tags

Gluten-free
Dairy-free
Vegan
Anti-inflammatory
No added refined sugar

Suggested cooking method/program

Stovetop, one-pot

Storage & meal prep tips

Store cooled golden milk in a sealed jar in the refrigerator for up to 3 days
Reheat gently on the stovetop, whisking to recombine before serving

Cortisol reset tip

Turmeric and cinnamon help lower inflammation and support healthy cortisol rhythms, while warm non-dairy milk and coconut oil promote relaxation for restful sleep

Possible variations

Add 1 teaspoon (5 ml) ashwagandha powder for extra adaptogenic support
Blend with 1 tablespoon (15 g) cashew butter for a creamier, more filling drink
Sprinkle with a pinch of ground nutmeg before serving for added sleep support. Use unsweetened coconut milk for a richer, tropical flavor.

79. Lemon-Ginger Cortisol-Calm Tea

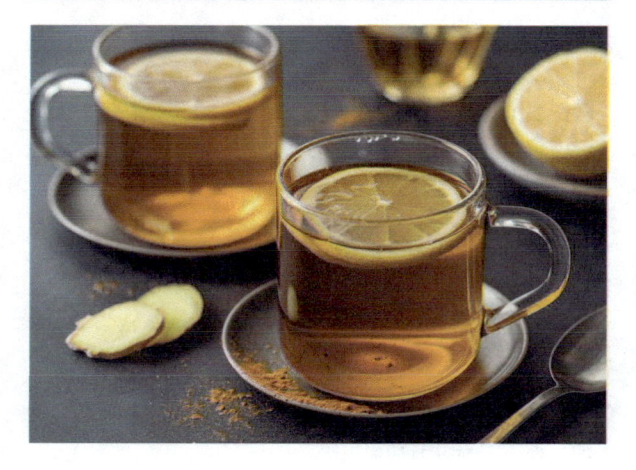

servings: 2

Ingredients

- 2 cups (480 ml) filtered water
- 1-inch (2.5 cm) piece fresh ginger, peeled and thinly sliced
- 1 organic lemon, sliced into rounds
- 1 tablespoon (15 ml) raw honey (optional, or use pure maple syrup for vegan)
- 1/4 teaspoon (1 g) ground turmeric (optional for extra anti-inflammatory boost)
- Pinch of ground black pepper (optional, enhances turmeric absorption)
- Optional swaps: Use lime instead of lemon; swap honey for monk fruit sweetener for low-sugar; omit black pepper for low-FODMAP

Directions

1. Add 2 cups (480 ml) filtered water and sliced ginger to a small saucepan
2. Bring to a gentle simmer over medium heat
3. Add lemon slices and optional turmeric and black pepper
4. Simmer uncovered for 5–7 minutes, until fragrant and slightly reduced
5. Remove from heat and strain into mugs
6. Stir in 1 tablespoon (15 ml) raw honey or sweetener of choice, adjusting to taste
7. Serve warm, garnished with extra lemon if desired

Estimated total time

Prep time: 3 minutes
Cook time: 7 minutes
Total: 10 minutes

Nutritional facts per serving

Calories: 30
Protein: 0 g
Fat: 0 g
Carbs: 8 g
Fiber: 1 g
Sugar: 6 g

Dietary labels/tags

Gluten-free
Dairy-free
Vegan-friendly (if using maple syrup)
Anti-inflammatory
Gentle-digestion

Suggested cooking method/program

Stovetop, one-pot

Storage & meal prep tips

Store cooled tea in a sealed glass jar in the refrigerator for up to 2 days
Reheat gently on the stovetop or enjoy chilled over ice

Cortisol reset tip

Ginger and lemon help reduce inflammation and support digestion, while the ritual of sipping warm tea can calm the nervous system and promote healthy cortisol balance

Possible variations

Add a few fresh mint leaves for a cooling effect. Steep with 1 green tea bag for a gentle energy lift
Use orange slices instead of lemon for a sweeter, less tart flavor Add 1/2 teaspoon (2.5 ml) ashwagandha powder for extra adaptogenic support

80. Cucumber-Mint Hydration Tonic with Aloe

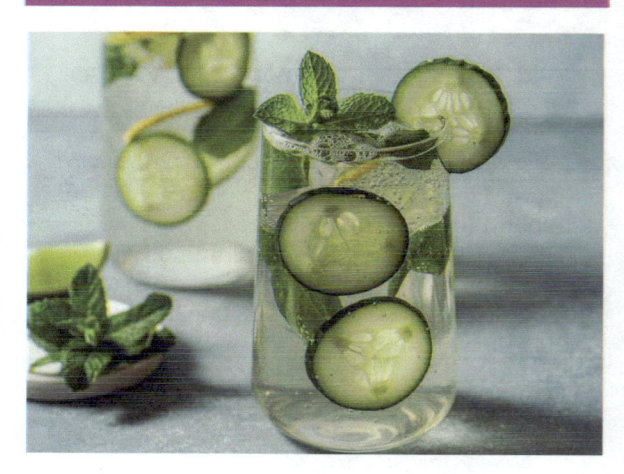

servings: 2

Ingredients

- 2 cups (480 ml) filtered water
- 1/2 large English cucumber (about 4 oz/115 g), thinly sliced
- 2 tablespoons (30 ml) pure aloe vera juice (food grade, inner fillet only)
- 6–8 fresh mint leaves
- 1 tablespoon (15 ml) fresh lime juice
- 1 teaspoon (5 ml) raw honey or pure maple syrup (optional, for gentle sweetness)
- Pinch of sea salt (about 1/16 teaspoon/0.3 g)
- Optional swaps: Use lemon juice instead of lime; swap honey for monk fruit sweetener for low-sugar; omit sweetener for Whole30; use coconut water instead of filtered water for extra electrolytes

Directions

1. Add 2 cups (480 ml) filtered water to a large glass jar or pitcher
2. Stir in 2 tablespoons (30 ml) aloe vera juice and 1 tablespoon (15 ml) fresh lime juice
3. Add 1/2 large cucumber (about 4 oz/115 g), thinly sliced, and 6–8 fresh mint leaves
4. Add 1 teaspoon (5 ml) raw honey or maple syrup, if using, and a pinch of sea salt
5. Stir well to combine, gently muddling the mint leaves with the back of a spoon to release flavor
6. Let sit for 5 minutes to infuse, or refrigerate up to 2 hours for a stronger flavor
7. Strain into glasses over ice, or serve as is with cucumber and mint for garnish

Estimated total time

Prep time: 5 minutes
No cook time
Total: 5 minutes

Nutritional facts per serving

Calories: 20
Protein: 0 g
Fat: 0 g
Carbs: 5 g
Fiber: 0 g
Sugar: 3 g

Dietary labels/tags

Gluten-free
Dairy-free
Vegan-friendly (if using maple syrup or monk fruit)
Anti-inflammatory
Gentle-digestion
Low-calorie

Suggested cooking method/program

No-cook, infusion

Storage & meal prep tips

Store in a sealed glass jar in the refrigerator for up to 24 hours
Stir before serving; best enjoyed fresh for optimal flavor and nutrient content

Cortisol reset tip

Aloe vera and cucumber soothe the digestive tract and help reduce inflammation, while mint and lime support hydration and gentle detox—key for balanced cortisol and energy

Possible variations

Add a few slices of fresh ginger for a subtle zing
Use sparkling water for a refreshing, bubbly tonic
Stir in 1/2 teaspoon (2.5 ml) chia seeds for extra fiber and satiety. Swap mint for fresh basil or cilantro for a different herbal note.

81. Berry-Lavender Nighttime Chamomile Infusion

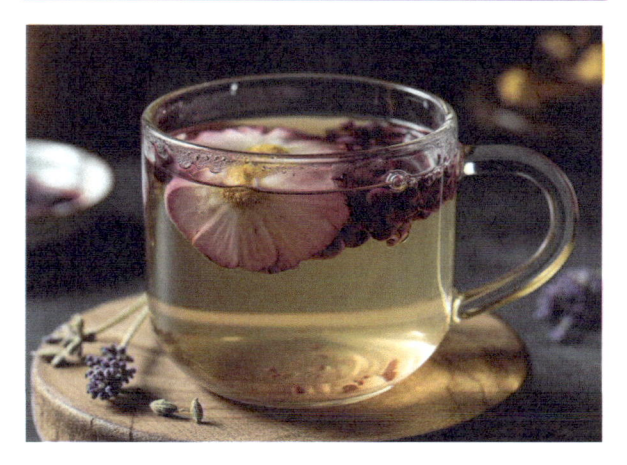

servings: 2

Ingredients

- 2 cups (480 ml) filtered water
- 2 chamomile tea bags (or 2 teaspoons/2 g loose dried chamomile flowers)
- 1/2 cup (75 g) fresh or frozen mixed berries (blueberries, raspberries, blackberries)
- 1/2 teaspoon (0.5 g) dried culinary lavender buds
- 1 teaspoon (5 ml) raw honey or pure maple syrup (optional, for gentle sweetness)

- 1/2 teaspoon (2.5 ml) fresh lemon juice (optional, for brightness)
- Optional swaps: Use all blueberries for a milder flavor; swap honey for monk fruit sweetener for low-sugar; omit lavender for low-FODMAP; use decaf green tea instead of chamomile for a different herbal note

Directions

1. Bring 2 cups (480 ml) filtered water to a gentle boil in a small saucepan or kettle
2. Add chamomile tea bags (or loose chamomile in a tea infuser), 1/2 cup (75 g) mixed berries, and 1/2 teaspoon (0.5 g) dried lavender buds to a large heatproof mug or teapot
3. Pour hot water over the ingredients
4. Cover and steep for 10 minutes to allow flavors and beneficial compounds to infuse
5. Remove tea bags and strain out berries and lavender using a fine mesh strainer
6. Stir in 1 teaspoon (5 ml) raw honey or maple syrup, and 1/2 teaspoon (2.5 ml) lemon juice if using
7. Serve warm, or let cool slightly and enjoy at room temperature

Estimated total time

Prep time: 5 minutes
Steep time: 10 minutes
Total: 15 minutes

Nutritional facts per serving

Calories: 25
Protein: 0 g
Fat: 0 g
Carbs: 6 g
Fiber: 1 g
Sugar: 4 g

Dietary labels/tags

Gluten-free
Dairy-free
Vegan-friendly (if using maple syrup or monk fruit)
Anti-inflammatory
Gentle-digestion
Caffeine-free

Suggested cooking method/program

Stovetop, infusion

Storage & meal prep tips

Store cooled infusion in a sealed glass jar in the refrigerator for up to 24 hours
Reheat gently or enjoy chilled; best consumed within 1 day for optimal flavor and potency

Cortisol reset tip

Chamomile and lavender promote relaxation and restful sleep, while berries provide antioxidants that help reduce inflammation and support overnight cortisol balance

Possible variations

Add a few fresh mint leaves for a cooling note
Use sliced strawberries for a sweeter, more floral infusion
Stir in 1/4 teaspoon (1.25 ml) ashwagandha powder for extra adaptogenic support. Swap lemon juice for orange zest for a different citrus twist

82. Apple Cider Detox Sparkler

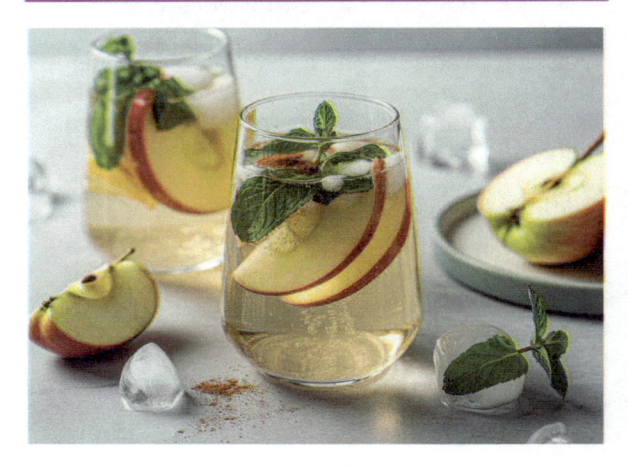

servings: 2

Ingredients

- 2 cups (480 ml) sparkling mineral water, chilled
- 2 tablespoons (30 ml) raw, unfiltered apple cider vinegar (with the "mother")
- 1 small crisp apple (about 5 oz/140 g), thinly sliced
- 1 tablespoon (15 ml) fresh lemon juice
- 1 teaspoon (5 ml) raw honey or pure maple syrup (optional, for gentle sweetness)
- 1/4 teaspoon (1 g) ground cinnamon
- 4–6 fresh mint leaves
- Pinch of sea salt (about 1/16 teaspoon/0.3 g)
- Optional swaps: Use monk fruit sweetener for low-sugar; swap lemon juice for lime; omit sweetener for Whole30; use still filtered water for a non-bubbly version

Directions

1. Add 2 tablespoons (30 ml) apple cider vinegar and 1 tablespoon (15 ml) fresh lemon juice to a large glass pitcher
2. Stir in 1 teaspoon (5 ml) raw honey or maple syrup, if using, and a pinch of sea salt
3. Add 1 small apple (about 5 oz/140 g), thinly sliced, and 4–6 fresh mint leaves
4. Sprinkle in 1/4 teaspoon (1 g) ground cinnamon
5. Pour in 2 cups (480 ml) chilled sparkling mineral water
6. Stir gently to combine, muddling the mint leaves and apple slices lightly with the back of a spoon
7. Let sit for 3–5 minutes to infuse flavors
8. Serve over ice, garnished with extra apple slices and mint if desired

Estimated total time

Prep time: 5 minutes
No cook time
Total: 5 minutes

Nutritional facts per serving

Calories: 20
Protein: 0 g
Fat: 0 g
Carbs: 5 g
Fiber: 1 g
Sugar: 3 g

Dietary labels/tags

Gluten-free
Dairy-free
Vegan-friendly (if using maple syrup or monk fruit)
Anti-inflammatory
Gentle-digestion
Low-calorie

Suggested cooking method/program

No-cook, infusion

Storage & meal prep tips

Best enjoyed fresh for optimal fizz and flavor
If prepping ahead, combine all ingredients except sparkling water and refrigerate up to 12 hours; add sparkling water just before serving
Store leftovers in a sealed glass jar in the refrigerator for up to 12 hours (may lose carbonation)

Cortisol reset tip

Apple cider vinegar and cinnamon help stabilize blood sugar and support healthy digestion, while lemon and mint provide gentle detoxification—key for balanced cortisol and reduced inflammation

Possible variations

Add a few thin slices of fresh ginger for a warming kick
Use pear slices instead of apple for a fall-inspired twist
Stir in 1/2 teaspoon (2.5 ml) chia seeds for extra fiber and satiety
Swap mint for fresh basil or rosemary for a different herbal note

REINTRODUCING FOODS SAFELY

After the initial 14–21 day reset phase, reintroducing foods requires careful attention because this stage helps identify specific sensitivities and shows how certain foods affect inflammation and cortisol. The goal is to add foods one at a time so you can monitor responses without overwhelming your system.

Start with a single item you missed during the reset — for example, *eggs*, *yogurt*, a slice of *sourdough*, or a serving of *beans*. Introduce only that one item so you can isolate its effects and spot any adverse reactions.

Begin with a small portion, about 2–3 bites, to lower the chance of a strong reaction and give your body time to adjust. Eat the reintroduced item at breakfast or lunch, ideally with a meal that includes protein and a variety of vegetables; this approach may help blunt spikes in cortisol and blood sugar while creating a steadier metabolic environment for digesting the new food.

Wait 48–72 hours before trying another new item. Use that interval to observe changes in your body and mood, and keep a detailed log tracking energy, mood, sleep, digestion, bloating, skin, joint pain, headaches, cravings, and resting morning pulse or heart rate variability.

If you notice symptoms within 0–72 hours after eating the food, record them carefully. Reactions can show up as digestive trouble, skin issues, mood shifts, or energy swings. Some people find that symptoms appear quickly, while others notice changes develop more gradually. If symptoms worsen, consider treating that food as **"not now"** and excluding it for another 4–8 weeks so your body can recover before a controlled retry.

This reintroduction process does more than reveal allergens or irritants; it teaches how specific foods interact with your system and helps you build a personalized eating plan. While some view this method as essential for identifying triggers, others prefer a less structured approach to dietary changes. Careful observation and consistent records can help you decide which items to keep and which to avoid.

Be patient and watchful—everyone's body reacts differently, and what works for someone else might not suit you. Some individuals find they can tolerate foods they previously avoided, while others discover new sensitivities they hadn't noticed before. Tune in to your signals and respond accordingly to create a diet that works for your unique needs.

On Day 1 of reintroducing a new food, offer a very small portion — about 2–3 bites (roughly 1 tablespoon) — to lower the risk of a strong allergic or intolerant reaction and let digestion adjust. If no adverse effects appear, on Day 2 increase to a moderate portion, typically 1/2 to 1 cup or a piece about the size of your palm, so you can better assess tolerance.

Keep all other meals low-reactive and anti-inflammatory during this two-day test: avoid introducing any other new items and stick to foods you already know work well for you. That isolation makes reactions easier to spot.

Consider starting with gentler preparations when possible. Some people find fermented dairy (*kefir* or *yogurt*) easier to tolerate than milk or cheese; others do better with soaked or sprouted legumes instead of regular canned or dry varieties; many prefer sourdough bread and steel-cut oats over commercial wheat products and instant oats. For eggs, testing pasture-raised eggs directly rather than in baked goods can provide clearer feedback, since these whole, minimally processed forms often digest more easily and offer a stronger nutrient profile.

Support the process with good sleep (**7–9 hours**), adequate hydration (about half your body weight in ounces daily), and soothing beverages like ginger or turmeric tea. A **10–20 minute walk after meals** aids digestion and steadies blood sugar. In the evening, magnesium can promote relaxation and better sleep; season food to taste with salt to help maintain sodium balance.

If a reaction occurs, follow the **reset triangle**: return to your baseline meals for 24 hours, increase fluids with electrolytes, and do one session of low-intensity movement (walking or gentle stretching) to help stabilize cortisol and allow recovery before trying the food

30-Day Cortisol Reset Meal Plan

(**B***: Breakfast | **L***: Lunch | **D***: Dinner | **S***: Snack)

PHASE 1 – CORTISOL CLEANSE (DAYS 1–7)

Day	Meals	Daily Focus Tip
1	**B:** Turmeric Chia Pudding with Berries **L:** Ginger-Turmeric Chicken Power Bowl **D:** Lemon-Garlic Turmeric Shrimp Skillet **S:** Turmeric Almond Energy Bites	Hydrate before breakfast to reduce cortisol.
2	**B:** Green Protein Smoothie with Spinach & Avocado **L:** Kale Quinoa Citrus Detox Salad **D:** Coconut-Ginger Tofu & Broccoli Stir-Skillet **S:** Lemon-Ginger Cortisol-Calm Tea	Walk outdoors for 10 minutes in the morning.
3	**B:** Golden Turmeric Oat Smoothie **L:** Mediterranean Chickpea & Kale Wrap **D:** One-Pot Lemon-Ginger Chicken with Quinoa & Kale **S:** Berry-Chia Lemon Cups	Add deep breathing before meals to aid digestion.
4	**B:** Smoked Salmon Avocado Rye Toast **L:** Warm Lentil Spinach Bowl with Walnuts **D:** Herbed Chicken Thighs with Zucchini & Olives **S:** Cucumber-Mint Hydration Tonic	Stretch lightly after lunch to support cortisol balance.
5	**B:** Cinnamon Walnut Quinoa Breakfast Bowl **L:** Avocado Hummus Veggie Wrap **D:** Sweet Potato, Kale & Lentil Hash with Tahini Drizzle **S:** Ginger-Date Walnut Bars	Aim for 7–8 hours of sleep tonight.
6	**B:** Berry Collagen Cortisol-Balance Smoothie **L:** Lemon-Tahini Salmon Grain Bowl **D:** Dijon Salmon with Asparagus & Sunflower Seeds **S:** Turmeric-Spiced Roasted Chickpeas	Practice gratitude journaling before bed.
7	**B:** Avocado Matcha Energy Shake **L:** Warm Quinoa, Roasted Chickpea & Walnut Power Plate **D:** Sheet Pan Turmeric Salmon with Roasted Fennel & Sweet Potato **S:** Lemon-Hemp Seed Kale Chips	Unplug from screens 1 hour before sleep.

PHASE 2 – GUT & INFLAMMATION RESET (DAYS 8–14)

Day	Meals	Daily Focus Tip
8	**B:** Berry-Kefir Overnight Oats with Flax **L:** Miso Mushroom & Baby Bok Choy Detox Soup **D:** Sheet Pan Harissa Eggplant with Chickpeas & Tahini **S:** Apple Cider Detox Sparkler	Chew slowly to improve digestion.
9	**B:** Almond Flour Blueberry Pancakes with Cinnamon **L:** Turmeric Lentil & Sweet Potato Soup **D:** Miso-Dijon Cod with Wilted Baby Spinach **S:** Ginger-Sesame Steamed Edamame	Drink water 30 minutes before meals.
10	**B:** Citrus-Ginger Hemp Yogurt Jar **L:** Mediterranean White Bean Stew with Kale & Olives **D:** One-Pot Coconut Miso Shrimp with Brown Rice & Baby Bok Choy **S:** Lemon-Ginger Cortisol-Calm Tea	Include a short walk after dinner.
11	**B:** Warm Hemp-Seed Porridge with Cinnamon & Pear **L:** Cucumber Mint Quinoa Tabbouleh with Pistachios **D:** Sheet Pan Herbed Turkey Meatballs with Brussels Sprouts & Cranberry Glaze **S:** Cortisol-Calm Apple Walnut Snack Packs	Take 5 deep breaths before each meal.
12	**B:** Sweet Potato Avocado Skillet with Poached Eggs **L:** Miso-Glazed Tempeh Lettuce Wraps with Ginger Slaw **D:** Lemon-Basil Turkey Cutlets with Sautéed Spinach **S:** No-Bake Almond-Cacao Energy Squares	Take a mindful pause mid-day.
13	**B:** Herbed Egg White Frittata with Asparagus & Sunflower Seeds **L:** Harissa-Lime Grilled Salmon with Zucchini Ribbons **D:** Coconut Curry Chickpea & Spinach Stew **S:** Berry-Lavender Nighttime Chamomile Infusion	Avoid caffeine after 2 PM.
14	**B:** Turmeric Spinach Egg Muffins **L:** Warm Farro with Roasted Brussels Sprouts & Pomegranate **D:** Herb-Crusted Baked Haddock with Roasted Fennel & Lemon **S:** Turmeric Almond Energy Bites	Take a warm bath to relax muscles.

PHASE 3 – HORMONE REBALANCE (DAYS 15–21)

Day	Meals	Daily Focus Tip
15	**B:** Avocado Soft-Boiled Eggs with Lemon Zest & Hemp Seeds **L:** Lemon-Dill Tuna & Cannellini Bean Plate with Arugula **D:** One-Pot Lemon-Ginger Chicken with Quinoa & Kale **S:** Sleep-Reset Turmeric Golden Milk	Get morning sunlight exposure.
16	**B:** Savory Spinach & Feta Egg Muffins with Pumpkin Seeds **L:** Miso-Maple Roasted Carrot & Lentil Bowl **D:** Cedar-Plank Lemon Trout with Steamed Asparagus **S:** Lemon-Ginger Cortisol-Calm Tea	Focus on protein at breakfast.
17	**B:** Almond-Butter Banana Chia Wrap **L:** Grilled Chicken, Avocado & Turmeric Slaw Wrap **D:** One-Pot Coconut Miso Shrimp with Brown Rice & Baby Bok Choy **S:** Ginger-Date Walnut Bars	Stretch for 5 minutes before bed.
18	**B:** Green Apple Spinach Detox Shake **L:** Herbed White Bean & Arugula Mason Jar Salad **D:** Sheet Pan Herbed Turkey Meatballs with Brussels Sprouts & Cranberry Glaze **S:** Cucumber-Mint Hydration Tonic with Aloe	Avoid eating 2 hours before sleep.
19	**B:** Warm Hemp-Seed Porridge with Cinnamon **L:** Black Bean Avocado & Mango Salad with Lime-Ginger Dressing **D:** Lemon-Basil Turkey Cutlets with Sautéed Spinach **S:** Turmeric-Spiced Roasted Chickpeas	Journal 3 wins before bed.
20	**B:** Almond Flour Blueberry Pancakes with Cinnamon **L:** Turmeric-Grilled Turkey, Avocado & Spinach Wrap **D:** Herb-Crusted Baked Haddock with Roasted Fennel & Lemon **S:** Berry-Lavender Nighttime Chamomile Infusion	Sleep 7+ hours tonight.
21	**B:** Sweet Potato & Apple Breakfast Hand Pies with Walnuts **L:** Mediterranean Eggplant, Quinoa & Walnut Lunch Bowl **D:** Miso-Glazed Tempeh & Broccoli Brown Rice Bowl **S:** Ginger-Sesame Steamed Edamame	Unplug during meals for mindful eating.

PHASE 4 – LONG-TERM ENERGY & BELLY FAT CONTROL (DAYS 22–30)

Day	Meals	Daily Focus Tip
22	**B:** Berry Collagen Cortisol-Balance Smoothie **L:** Kale Quinoa Citrus Detox Salad **D:** Sheet Pan Turmeric Salmon with Roasted Fennel & Sweet Potato **S:** Lemon-Ginger Cortisol-Calm Tea	Drink lemon water in the morning.
23	**B:** Golden Turmeric Oat Smoothie **L:** Warm Lentil Spinach Bowl with Walnuts **D:** One-Pot Lemon-Ginger Chicken with Quinoa & Kale **S:** Turmeric Almond Energy Bites	Add short mindful breathing breaks.
24	**B:** Green Protein Smoothie with Spinach & Avocado **L:** Cucumber Mint Quinoa Tabbouleh with Pistachios **D:** Cedar-Plank Lemon Trout with Steamed Asparagus **S:** Lemon-Hemp Seed Kale Chips	Avoid sugar after dinner.
25	**B:** Turmeric Spinach Egg Muffins **L:** Harissa-Lime Grilled Salmon with Zucchini Ribbons **D:** Coconut Curry Chickpea & Spinach Stew **S:** Sleep-Reset Turmeric Golden Milk	Do gentle yoga or stretching.
26	**B:** Herbed Egg White Frittata with Asparagus & Sunflower Seeds **L:** Miso Mushroom & Baby Bok Choy Detox Soup **D:** Lemon-Dill Tuna & Cannellini Bean Plate with Arugula **S:** Ginger-Date Walnut Bars	Stay hydrated all day.
27	**B:** Green Apple Spinach Detox Shake **L:** Warm Farro with Roasted Brussels Sprouts & Pomegranate **D:** One-Pot Coconut Miso Shrimp with Brown Rice & Baby Bok Choy **S:** Turmeric Almond Energy Bites	Practice gratitude before bed.
28	**B:** Avocado Matcha Energy Shake **L:** Mediterranean Chickpea & Kale Wrap **D:** Herb-Crusted Baked Haddock with Roasted Fennel & Lemon **S:** Berry-Lavender Nighttime Chamomile Infusion	Go tech-free 30 minutes before bed.
29	**B:** Almond-Butter Banana Chia Wrap **L:** Lemon-Tahini Salmon Grain Bowl **D:** Herbed Chicken Thighs with Zucchini & Olives **S:** Lemon-Ginger Cortisol-Calm Tea	Focus on slow, calm eating.
30	**B:** Sweet Potato Avocado Skillet with Poached Eggs **L:** Black Bean Avocado & Mango Salad with Lime-Ginger Dressing **D:** Sheet Pan Herbed Turkey Meatballs with Brussels Sprouts & Cranberry Glaze **S:** No-Bake Almond-Cacao Energy Squares	Celebrate your progress and set new goals.

Conclusion

In a balanced, anti-inflammatory lifestyle, keep things simple and be kind to yourself. Aim to follow your core **green-meal template** and **protein-forward anchors** while preserving **cortisol-friendly rhythms** about 80–90% of the time. This approach allows you to stay flexible without guilt, accept life's unpredictability, and avoid chasing perfection. While some prefer stricter adherence, others find that this framework helps build a sustainable routine that supports health goals while accommodating inevitable variations.

Review your **food–symptom log** monthly, tracking what you eat and how your body reacts in different situations. Consider celebrating one measurable win each month—better sleep, more energy, or less bloating—to reinforce progress and identify areas to refine. Focus on a single change at a time, whether increasing protein, adding steps to your day, improving sleep, or sharpening stress-management skills. Small, steady tweaks tend to accumulate and boost overall well-being.

Make a relapse-ready plan by choosing three reliable baseline meals you can count on during hard moments. Keep these meals simple, nutritious, and satisfying so they meet your body's needs. You might pair that with a 10-minute walk plus breathwork to help lower cortisol and calm your system. Also consider keeping a short *"calm kitchen"* restock list so you always have basic ingredients for quick, healthy meals.

When setbacks hit—PMS, travel, or tight deadlines—returning to your baseline meals for 24–72 hours can help your body recalibrate and feel steadier. During that time, prioritizing hydration and sleep while pausing food reintroductions until stress levels drop may allow your body to better process new foods.

Made in United States
Cleveland, OH
06 November 2025